"I had no idea how much my life would change in only a month. With SHRED I'm down a total of twenty-seven pounds. At my age and metabolism, this is a miracle. I am a SHREDDER for life." —Beverly

"Thank you for SHRED! I've lost for good, five pounds during the first week. SHRED ROCKS!" — Renita

"This has been the best lifestyle change!" —Jenell

"@doctoriansmith has me under his spell." —Tawnya

"Workout done! 1,194 cals burned! Day twelve of #Shred. Giving 110 percent. Lost five pounds last week. Can't wait to see scale Mon." —Nicole

"Week one I lost 7.6 pounds . . . Excited! I went an entire week without any soda!" —Sheree

"Dr. Ian is a miracle worker! Couldn't believe my scale this morning." —Melissa

"I was able to handle my meals and not overeat when I went to the game tonight. This is huge for me because I usually can't resist stadium food. Victory one for me came tonight!" —Justin

SHRED

The Revolutionary Diet

6 WEEKS

4 INCHES

2 SIZES

Ian K. Smith, M.D.

St. Martin's Paperbacks

SHRED: THE REVOLUTIONARY DIET

Copyright © 2012 by Ian K. Smith, M.D.

All rights reserved.

For information address St. Martin's Press, 175 Fifth Avenue, New York, NY 10010.

EAN: 978-1-250-08051-6

Printed in the United States of America

St. Martin's Press edition / January 2013
St. Martin's Griffin edition / May 2014
St. Martin's Paperbacks edition / January 2016

St. Martin's Paperbacks are published by St. Martin's Press, 175 Fifth Avenue, New York, NY 10010.

10 9 8 7 6 5 4 3 2 1

I dedicate this book to my grandfather, Robert S. Cherry, Sr. Even in his ninth decade of life, he continues to love, inspire, motivate, educate, and humble me. I love you, Pops. You have been the always reliable foundation of my very existence.

Note to the Reader

Contents

Acknowledgments

Any author will tell you that while his or her name is on the cover of a book, there are many people's names that don't make it but who deserve special recognition, as their contributions are superbly integral to the entire process. Most likely you will not recognize the following names, but all are extremely significant to me and the book you are about to read. They are listed in no particular order other than the whimsy of my recalling them. This final product in different ways is a testament to each of them: Tristé Smith, Dashiell Smith, Declan Smith, Dana Smith, Liza Rodriguez, Rena Cherry, Jonathan Cardi, Ron Mitchell, Michael Strahan, Rebecca Casey, Maritza Villalobos, Elizabeth Beier, Michelle Richter, Steve Cohen, Matthew Shear, Sally Richardson, John Karle, John Murphy, Michael Storrings, Kerri Resnick, Pam El, Don Arbuckle, Ojinika Obiekwe, Edgar Quijano. A special thanks to all of the SHREDDERs who are part of shredder Nation (www.facebook.com/Shredder Nation) and who gave me their feedback on the diet early in the process, losing lots of weight, and making many useful suggestions that I have incorporated in this final version of the plan.

Introduction

This book came about by accident, and like many great things in life that arrive in this manner, it was destiny not to be denied. I was working with a friend who I had helped lose weight in the past. She had dropped nearly 30 percent of her body weight in approximately eighteen months. She looked great, felt great, and was doing things physically that she hadn't been able to do since she was in high school. However, she started to become frustrated because she couldn't drop the last twenty pounds that would take her to her ultimate goal. Dejected, she called me and asked me if there was anything I could do to help.

My first instinct was that there was nothing left to do except for her to work harder, exercise more, maybe take in fewer calories—standard weight-loss stuff. You know it. I know it. We all know it. But then I looked back at some of her food and exercise journals as well as my previous books, which I'd given her and which had brought her tremendous success. Sitting at my desk and looking through it all sparked several thoughts. She was in need of something different and out of the box. Her body had become accustomed to all of the good habits she had developed. Her success, ironically, was keeping her from *more* success. So I got the idea to create a program that used all that I knew about strategic dieting and combined it in one plan. It would be like taking your best players on a team and putting them out on the field at once to maximize your chance of winning a game. I immediately went to work and over the next couple of weeks formulated the foundation of a plan that I thought would kick-start her metabolism and help her break through this frustrating plateau. I also decided to give the plan a name that would be demonstrative of what she would be doing, an action word so that every time she looked at it or heard it, her mind would visualize what was going on internally as she followed the program: SHRED. This was all about shredding that stubborn fat.

She did great on the plan. She was able to break through the plateau and get on the path to ultimate success. I'm always trying to learn, so I asked her for detailed feedback and criticisms of the program—what was too difficult, what she liked, what would make it better, etc. Over the next year I kept working on SHRED, and as various friends came to me and asked for help that could take them beyond the advice in my other diet books, which they had already tried successfully, I'd dust off the latest version of SHRED and send it to them. Each time the results were the same. They lost weight immediately and the dreaded plateau was in their rearview mirror. SHRED had become my secret weapon.

Realizing that there were millions out there struggling with those pockets of stubborn fat, I decided to start a challenge on Twitter. I would tweet daily diet tips from SHRED to my followers (my Twitter handle is @doctoriansmith). It wasn't easy doing this in just 140 characters, but I truncated and abbreviated and found a way to get the messages across. The results practically knocked me off my feet. My followers were losing significant amounts of weight in a short period of time, some as much as 10 pounds in just one week; before I knew it, thousands of people were on the program and they were SHRED-DING fat like they never had before on any other program. They told me this was the first plan that brought them consistent and at times dramatic weight loss, and they still felt as though they had enough to eat. In some cases, I even heard complaints that SHREDDING involved too much food. What a problem to have!

These first SHREDDERs not only found success on the scale, but the program was life altering for them in many other ways. They sent me e-mails saying that they were more confident and determined and had energy levels they hadn't had in years. They felt like new people. Life was suddenly a new adventure for them. Most telling was that *all* of them who wrote me were determined never to return to the old life and habits they had left behind. This new way of living was so much more fun and promising. It felt great!

SHREDDERs have sprouted up across the country and as far away as the United Kingdom. Hearing their successes and gratitude for the plan has been the biggest reward for me. No diet is perfect and there's no one program that will work for everyone. But I truly believe that whether it's weight lost, inches eliminated, or sizes dropped, everyone can benefit from SHREDDING. It's not a diet—it's a way of life! Welcome to SHREDDER Nation. Believe! Work hard! Have fun!

For free weight-loss and other health tips,
follow Dr. Ian on Twitter: @doctoriansmith;
or on his Web site: www.doctoriansmith.com;
or on his Facebook page:
www.facebook.com/ShredderNation

CHAPTER 1

The SHRED Concept

SHRED is a revolutionary diet plan that combines several different strategies in an effort to help users lose weight, increase confidence, and improve overall wellness. Unlike many other programs that simply focus on how many pounds are lost on the scale, SHRED also improves other health factors, such as reducing risk for high blood pressure, decreasing the risk for diabetes, and improving energy levels. With so many programs available it is reasonable to ask why one would choose SHRED over another popular diet. The answer is simple. SHRED allows you to eat normal food that's inexpensive. It is extremely simple to understand, and it does not require perfection for you to find success. Another important aspect that many SHREDDERs have liked is that the diet can be customized based on the results you're looking for or any dietary preferences you might have. You will find that making substitutions while SHREDDING is not only allowed but encouraged, as it will not impede your success in any way.

There are many programs that can help you lose weight, but there are few that combine the appropriate balance of challenging you while at the same time not making it too difficult to follow for the long term. One major problem with many diet plans is that while they can help users lose weight, they are so extreme, difficult, or uncomfortable that dieters are unable to follow the guidelines for an extended period of time. The second you stop following the plan, the pounds that were lost pile back on with a vengeance, and often, then some. This is not the case with SHRED. The vast majority of those surveyed who tried the early versions of the program repeatedly commented that unlike other plans they had tried, SHRED was one they could see themselves following forever.

There are many principles at work in SHRED that lead to the tremendous success that so many experience. Ease of use is at the top of the list: each day is thoughtfully planned out so that your need to think about what works and what doesn't is kept to a minimum. Ironically, many who have been asked about programs that give them the greatest level of flexibility in choosing the foods they can eat say that too much flexibility can actually make the diet more difficult. It's a struggle to have so many choices in front of them. SHRED spells out in detail each meal you will consume for six weeks, but it also gives you plenty of room to make substitutions so that you can swap out meals if you like.

SHRED is a six-week program. You may well stay on SHRED for more than six weeks, but each six weeks is considered to be a cycle. Based on the hundreds of SHREDDERs who have tried the program and provided feedback, the average weight loss for a cycle is between 18 and 25 pounds. Results, as with any diet program, will vary from person to person for various reasons, but more than with any diet I've developed or been aware of, what has been amazingly satisfying is how consistent the weight loss has been. Ninety-three percent of the people who have been on the program have lost weight each week of the cycle. Even better, many who had been using other diet plans and had hit a plateau found that just a *week* on SHRED got them losing weight again.

In general, those who are closer to their target weight will definitely lose weight but tend to lose weight a little more slowly. This is to be expected, so if you fall into this category, don't be disappointed if you don't see the numbers on the scale drop quickly or significantly at first. Look for any progress, whether it be increased energy or losing inches. However, those who have more than 30 pounds to lose will typically start seeing results right away. The average results on SHRED are 6-4-2. In six weeks most people who closely follow the program lose four inches and two sizes.

Once you have completed an initial six-week cycle, if you still have more weight to lose, the program is designed for you to cycle again. After the first cycle, you can reorder the weeks of a new cycle in any fashion that works best for you. This is only one way in which SHRED can be customized to fit your needs. I recognize that there's no such thing as "one size fits all" when it comes to diet plans, but SHRED comes close.

SHRED CYCLES

Each week of SHRED is designed to stand on its own and to be different from the weeks before. Each of the six weeks has a name that reflects the theme for that week. The weeks are Prime, Challenge, Transformation, Ascend, Cleanse, and Explode. While each week represents a leg in your journey, it also builds on those that precede it. The program teaches you how to make smarter choices and has specific strategies embedded in the daily meal and exercise plans: sometimes you will recognize them and other times you will not. The overall effect, however, is that you will continuously SHRED fat. You will see the declining numbers on the scale and a reduction in inches wherever you need to lose them: whether it be in your waist, thighs, or hips.

It has been my experience that programs that start out asking followers to make extreme changes in their dietary and/or exercise habits are least effective over the long term. Users either can never fully engage the program, because it's asking too much of them, or they are able to do some of the program but not all of it, leading them to become discouraged and drop out altogether. SHRED acknowledges some very basic facts. First, losing weight is not easy and quite often is extremely frustrating. Second, no one is a perfect eater or exerciser and expecting someone—anyone—to be perfect and not have bad days is completely unrealistic. Third, success comes from following a program that one can ease into, rather than a program that starts out too aggressively rigorous and restrictive. People don't always want to feel like they're on a diet!

Prime. These seven days prime you for the rest of the plan. This week is an induction into SHREDDER Nation. You'll learn about the importance of meal spacing, proper snacking techniques, and suppressing hunger without consuming too many calories. The average weight loss this week will be 3.5 pounds. This could be less if you're within 20 pounds of your goal weight. The further you are away from your target weight and the worse your habits have been prior to starting the program, the more weight you will lose. Many who fit this description have lost as much as 8 to 10 pounds during Prime. One hundred percent of the people who have been on the program—regardless of how much weight they needed to lose—answered in their survey that they had enough to eat, some going so far as to say that there was *so* much food they couldn't manage to eat everything on the daily menus.

Challenge is a week that asks you to demand more of yourself. It asks you to release some of your bad habits and adopt some new behaviors that you will have for the rest of your life. This week says that you can do better: you'll learn after a couple of days that despite early doubts you might have about yourself, you actually can rise to the challenge. This week is a confidence booster, because it shows many dieters that despite their failures in the past or what they have previously perceived to be difficult, they actually have what it takes to succeed. At the end of the Challenge you will be motivated more than ever to truly make a commitment to a healthier lifestyle and to reach the goals you have set forth prior to starting your SHRED.

Transformation week is a critical seven days where most SHREDDERs start truly noticing a difference. Not only will the scale reflect your hard work, but many realize for the first time at the end of this week that they have dropped a clothing size, their energy levels are much greater, and their outlook about their success on the program heightens dramatically. Transformation is designed to be the toughest week of the program. You will be challenged the most during this week, but it's nothing you can't handle. Knowing this week is the toughest is half the battle. The other half is putting your head down and getting through it. If you focus, this week will be your best friend. Every day visualize the fat being SHREDDED and your body's appearance changing.

Ascend is an important turnaround week. Imagine that for the last three weeks you have been descending into a pit. Last week you finally reached the bottom and started to regain strength so that you can climb your way out. The seven days of Ascend have been specifically constructed so that you are now exiting the darkness and ascending toward the light. You have already completed the toughest week of the program, so Ascend will come as a relief. You will continue to work hard, but the work will not feel as strenuous as it did the week before. Re-invigorated after three weeks on the program, you are now energized to finish the rest of the cycle at full speed.

Cleanse is a week that pays special attention to enhancing your liver's ability to detoxify your blood. All of us—even those who eat as healthfully as possible—accumulate some level of toxins in our bodies. We want to eliminate these toxins as efficiently as possible. Sometimes livers can be overwhelmed, so occasionally it's beneficial to give them a little boost in carrying out their jobs. Certain foods can provide this boost by activating special enzymes in the liver that facilitate the cleansing process. There are also foods that work to increase the activity of the gastrointestinal tract. This creates a physical cleanse. This week you will do both. Not only will you improve your physical health this week, but you will continue your weight loss: some will lose their largest amounts during these seven days.

Explode is the last week of the cycle. It's meant to help you end the cycle with a bang. For some, this week will be their last and they will have reached their goal. For others, Explode is a launching pad into the next cycle. At this point in the program SHREDDERs will have gone through the toughest as well as the easiest portions of the cycle and now are using all they have learned to explode into a new lifestyle that will serve them well for the rest of their lives. The purpose of SHRED is not only to get rid of excess weight and the bad habits that have contributed to the problem, but to position you so that you no longer have to be on a diet. No longer will you need to read the plan or follow the meal plans to the letter; you will now be eating, drinking, and exercising in a manner that you can do for the rest of your life.

MEAL SPACING

A lot is made in every diet about what you eat, how much you eat, and how many calories you consume. These three factors, of course, have a tremendous impact on whether the body will gain weight, maintain weight, or lose weight. But a factor that is lost on many people is the spacing of meals. Research has continuously shown that spacing your meals and snacks in a regular manner can be extremely advantageous to weight loss. Hormones such as insulin and cortisol play a role in weight gain and, subsequently, weight loss. New research has shown that keeping hormone levels as consistent as possible and avoiding spikes in their release and, their concentration in blood levels can be an added benefit when dieting.

SHRED pays as much attention to *when* you're eating as it does to what you're eating. Throughout the six weeks, the plan guides you to strategically time your meals. Everyone understands the relationship between calorie counts and weight gain, but for many it might come as a new concept that the timing of your meals and snacks can be a reason why you are or aren't losing weight. Many of us have extremely irregular and unhealthy eating schedules: SHRED can get you on a routine that will not only help you lose weight, but prevent you from having those intense bouts of hunger between meals.

DIET CONFUSION

We can learn a lot from the world of weight lifting. There's a well-known principle when it comes to lifting weights called "muscle confusion." Not everyone believes in this principle, but it has its ardent supporters and has been around for a long time. I find it to be an interesting principle. The basis of muscle confusion is that if one performs the same exercise—let's say for two months your workout regimen involves lifting five-pound dumbbells every other day for ten repetitions per set for three sets. After a period of time, your muscles start to accommodate to the exercise. This means that the more often your muscles perform this routine, the more efficient they become at it. The more efficient they become at performing the exercise, the more likely you are to plateau and not burn as many calories. Basically, the muscles are no longer impressed or stressed enough by the exercise because they have seen it too often for too long, and so they know what to expect and how to best deal with it. They no longer need to expend the same relative effort that was required when you first started the exercise routine. The more you do the exercise the less of a return you get for your efforts.

The theory of muscle confusion says that it's possible to confuse the muscles and prevent a plateau by varying the types of exercises, sets, repetitions, and weights. So instead of using the dumbbells in the same fashion every time you work out, try a different machine, a different amount of weight, or a different number of repetitions. The belief is that if you do this you will continue to challenge the muscles and optimize growth and caloric burn.

While this theory typically applies to muscle growth, SHRED adopts a similar theoretical approach when it comes to nutrition. The idea is that by eating the same food all of the time, a couple of things can happen. First, there's an increased chance that you will reach diet boredom. At some point you will tire of eating the same thing and the temptation to eat something that's not on the plan increases to the point where you start sampling off the menu. One small sampling leads to bigger sampling, until eventually you are barely following the plan and making up your own rules as you see fit. The second thing that could theoretically happen is that by eating the same food all of the time, the body becomes acclimated to eating those foods and more efficient at processing them. This increased efficiency means less energy needed for digestion. So varying your nutritional choices can keep the body guessing, and it's this guessing that could keep up your metabolism and keep your body off kilter. SHRED introduces a variety of foods in the hopes of decreasing your chances of food boredom and possibly increasing your metabolism.

THE SHREDDER MENTALITY

Dieting is 80 percent mental and 20 percent physical. Why is it that two people who have the same plan to follow can have such different results or levels of engagement? Why can some people who do the work to lose weight keep off the pounds, but others who have also succeeded end up gaining them back? Why do some people give up after only a couple of weeks on a plan, even though they are experiencing success? In many cases, one's mentality is a large part of these answers. The mental aspect of dieting can never be overstated. Willpower, discipline, motivation—these are universally mentioned by the vast majority of dieters who say they have tried to lose weight in the past, but have not been successful. Regardless of how good a plan might be, if one doesn't believe in it and follow it, success will not be achieved. SHRED has built-in strategies that grow confidence and keep you inspired to stick with the plan and achieve success. In fact, many are so concentrated on the food and exercise as they are going through the cycle, they don't even realize they are also developing the mental toughness critical for success.

Many programs penalize users if they stray from the plan or don't give 100 percent. SHRED will never do this. SHRED is what I like to call a forgiving plan. SHRED understands that no one can eat or exercise perfectly, so it never requires or expects it. Many who have followed the plan have sent me e-mails expressing confidence that they will never return to the bad habits that put them in the difficult predicament from which they have finally emerged. They often speak about how for the first time, after many failed dieting attempts, they now have the willpower to do what they have always known is the right thing to do. SHREDDERs develop a new mental approach not just to food, beverages, and exercise, but also to the entirety of life.

CHAPTER 2

How SHRED Works

SHRED is one of the easiest programs to deliver a high level of results. My job is to take complicated weight-loss principles and distill them down to simple strategies that are easy to implement. You will not have to overthink anything you do while SHREDDING. The first time you go through the six-week cycle, you will do so in the exact order I've laid out. There are many reasons why I've ordered the sequence the way I have. To achieve maximum success, strictly adhering to the order is advised.

Each week is laid out for you in detail. All you need to do is follow the meals and, if necessary, make substitutions. Chapters 9, 10, 11, and 12 contain more than two hundred snacks and more than fifty recipes for smoothies, shakes, and soups. You can use my suggestions or find your own. The key, however, is to make sure whatever you consume falls into the guidelines as laid out in the beginning of each week and those within the daily plan.

CYCLING

Each cycle consists of six weeks, but many of you will need to do more than one cycle of SHRED in order to achieve your goals. This is completely expected: I have written the program so that this can be done most effectively. While the sequence of weeks is critical during the first cycle of SHRED, subsequent cycles can be customized so that they make the most sense to your schedule and particular needs. For SHRED to work best for you, it's important during the first cycle that you keep brief notes as you go through the weeks. You should record what you find difficult about the week, what you find easy, and ultimately how much you lose during that seven-day period. This information is important, because if you decide to do a second cycle, you can then arrange the weeks strategically. Let's say that week 3, Transformation, is the week in which you lost the most weight. Let's also say that week 2, Challenge, is the one that you felt worked the best as far as your ability to stick to the plan and at the same time lose weight. It's possible that week 4, Ascend, gave you the second greatest weight loss. You've finished the entire six-week cycle and you still have 8 pounds left before you reach your goal. This means it's unlikely you will need to do the entire six-week cycle again, but you'll need somewhere between two and three weeks to get off the final pounds. Now is when those notes you took can make a difference: look back at them and see which weeks worked best for you. In our example, this would be weeks 2, 3, and 4. So while you decide how you do your next cycle, instead of starting with week 1, you could start with either weeks 2, 3, or 4 and work through them to achieve the 8-pound loss that you're hoping to achieve. If these three weeks are not enough to knock off the final 8 pounds, you can always go on and redo other weeks of the cycle.

For those who have 25 pounds or less to lose, you can start with week 1 in the cycle, but don't be surprised if you don't see large results early on. Prime week really is about getting you organized for the next five weeks, and while others will lose 3 to 5 pounds even while priming, you might only see minimal weight loss. Don't be discouraged in the least. This is completely normal and has no bearing on your potential success during the rest of the cycle. You should really see progress in week 2, Challenge. Because you begin closer to your target weight than most, your adherence to the guidelines of the program is critical for fast and optimal results. Because you don't have a significant amount of weight to lose compared to many others—who might have 40 pounds or more—your margin of error is narrower. Don't be discouraged, but be inspired to really give it your all. While it won't hurt you to start your cycle with week 1, you can also skip Prime and go right to week 2.

EXERCISING

SHRED is not only about what you eat, but how you move. The exercise requirement for each day is spelled out just the way the daily menus are. There is no doubt that you can lose significant weight just by following the menus and making the dietary choices the plan recommends, but you should be looking for more than that. Exercise is critical for maximizing weight loss. This is what SHREDDING is all about. Better nutritional choices and exercise are a one-two punch when it comes to weight loss. But beyond the number on the scale, exercise is critical for overall wellness. Building lean muscle mass through resistance training will increase your metabolism, which in turn increases how many calories your body burns. Exercise is important to strengthen your bones, improve blood flow, reduce your risk for diabetes, reduce your risk for heart diseases, and increase balance and flexibility.

When the plan calls for a certain amount of exercise for that day, the plan also gives you flexibility in how you complete it. For example, until you get accustomed to exercising on a regular basis, rather than trying to do all of the recommended daily exercise at once, you should consider breaking it up into two sessions. If, let's say, the exercise requirement is 40 minutes, but you don't have time to complete it all at once or your endurance is not equal to accomplishing it all in one session, feel free to break the workout up into two 20-minute sessions that day. The key is not just the amount of exercise you do, but the intensity of the exercise. Stop pretending that exercising will not deliver any benefits and is simply a waste of time. You need to get your heart rate up and perform at a moderate level of intensity. If you can complete the exercise for any given day in a more intense manner, then you will achieve your goals faster.

The first cycle of SHRED requires only that you participate in cardio. This is by design. Don't interpret this as meaning that resistance training (lifting free weights, weight machines, using resistance bands) is a bad thing.

Quite the contrary. In fact, after you do the first SHRED cycle, I recommend that you add weight lifting or some other type of resistance training to your regimen. Building lean muscle mass increases your metabolism, which in turn helps you burn more calories throughout the day. Resistance training has other health benefits, too, such as improving blood flow, increasing bone density and strength, improving mobility and balance, and preventing medical conditions such as diabetes, heart disease, and arthritis.

Those who do more than one cycle should begin resistance training during the second cycle. If you are inexperienced, take lessons from a certified professional so you can be sure you are doing the exercises safely and effectively. The resistance training should not replace your cardio. Instead, do 20 minutes of resistance work 2 to 3 times per week in addition to the cardio. Simply add it to your cardio workout or choose to do it during your rest days. Whatever you prefer is fine, as long as you're able to get it in. Resistance training will help increase your muscle tone and sculpt your body.

SUBSTITUTIONS

Great effort and thought has gone into the structure of SHRED. Beyond what scientific research has shown, early feedback from thousands who have tried the program has informed the plan in this book. This, however, doesn't make the plan perfect, nor does it mean there aren't things that can be modified on an individual basis to improve its effectiveness. Unlike other plans that don't allow one letter of a plan to be changed, SHRED actually allows flexibility. You might have allergies, taste preferences, access issues, medical conditions, etc., that prevent you from eating or drinking a particular food or beverage. SHRED allows you to make substitutions for these items. It's important, however, to make *smart* substitutions. If you don't eat meat and the meal option is a meat, then obviously you need to make a switch. Fish or a salad are great substitution options; three slices of triple-cheese pizza is not.

It's impossible for any diet plan to think of every possible scenario or consider every food manufacturer and their products. Just because something's not mentioned doesn't mean it isn't allowed; just use good judgment and try to make smart decisions. Part of becoming a SHREDDER is becoming a good decision maker. You are going to be faced with food choices for the rest of your life, whether at a friend's barbecue or a restaurant you might visit on family vacation. You will not always have this book to guide you through your selection. Once you learn the SHRED philosophy and get an understanding of smart choices, you will be able to eat anywhere and feel comfortable that you can enjoy yourself while staying lean and healthy.

MAINTENANCE

Reaching your weight-loss goal is not the only important accomplishment when you become a SHREDDER.

After initial weight loss, the issue you face is maintaining that weight loss. It's critical as you go through the cycle(s) that you start adopting as many of the eating and exercising behaviors in SHRED as possible and permanently leave behind some of the poor choices and lifestyle behaviors that contributed to your original weight problems. The true success of SHREDDING comes after a while, when SHREDDING becomes such a way of life for you that you no longer even need to check the plan to make sure you're on track. You are now making smarter choices—not perfect, but smarter. Once you have reached your goal, you are ready for maintenance. So, once a month you should choose a SHRED week and stick to that week vigilantly, following the menus and exercises as written. This is like giving your car a tune-up. You take your car to a mechanic for a tune-up not because it's not working properly, but because it's wiser to get parts serviced and tested periodically so that if something is heading toward dysfunction, you can catch it early when the fix is cheaper and easier. Waiting too long is costly, inconvenient, and a bigger headache. Your SHRED tune-up is strictly following a week of your choice—not the same each time—once a month. After six months of maintaining your weight loss, you can move this tune-up to once every two months.

Now let's get busy. It's time to SHRED!

CHAPTER 3

Week 1: Prime

This is the first leg of your journey. For some, Prime will be a radically different way of eating and exercising, while for others it will be only slightly different from what they've already been doing. This week will prime you for success as you go through the rest of the plan. It will set up the weeks that follow, so pay close attention to the timing of your meals, making sure that you eat them about every three to four hours. Your snacks—if you chose to have them—will come between the meals, but no sooner than an hour after eating a meal. You can refer to chapter 9 for a selection of more than two hundred snacks, chapter 10 for smoothie recipes, chapter 11 for protein shake recipes, and chapter 12 for sample soup recipes. You are not obligated to use these lists or recipes; they are there for your convenience and can be extremely helpful as you SHRED.

Timing is critical to the success of this plan. It might be difficult at first, but plan in advance and do the best you can. Skipping meals is not advised. Even if you eat just a small portion, try to eat something on schedule. A sample day's schedule during Prime might look something like the grid below, but for each and every day, the order of the meals and snacks is both intended and critical. And on some days, there's a bonus fourth snack, so follow each day's directions carefully.

8:30 A.M.	10:00 A.M.	11:30 A.M.	1:00 P.M.	3:30 P.M.	7:00 P.M.	8:30 P.M.
Meal 1	Snack 1	Meal 2	Snack 2	Meal 3	Meal 4	Snack 3

While you might be anxious to jump right into the program, it's critical that you read the week's guidelines first. They will fill in holes you might encounter and answer the questions that you'll inevitably have. Substitutions can be made on this program, but make them wisely and selectively. Try your best to stick to the plan as it is laid out. Believe! Work hard! Have fun!

SHRED WEEK 1 GUIDELINES

▶ Weigh yourself in the morning before starting the program and record it. Don't weigh yourself throughout the week. Your next weigh-in will be the same day the following week in the morning. Weigh yourself in the same manner as you did in the beginning. If you weighed in without wearing clothes initially, then do that again. If you weighed in wearing certain clothes, wear the same clothes for the second weigh-in. Use the same scale both times. *Don't* use a different scale as scales can differ by several pounds.

▶ You must eat something every 3 to 4 hours even if you're not hungry, but *don't* stuff yourself. Eat until you're no longer hungry, but *don't eat until you're full*. If you need less than what's recommended, then great, go ahead and eat less, which is even better. If you want to switch meals, that is permitted, but try to switch as infrequently as possible. For example, if you know that what's listed for meal 3 is easier to get than what's listed for meal 2, then go ahead and switch them. Looking at the day's meals in advance is important as it allows you to best prepare for what's ahead. Remember, the meals are every 3 to 4 hours and the snacks come between the meals. Snacks are not a meal.

▶ Five out of the seven days you must do cardiovascular exercise, commonly called cardio. Pay attention to the guidelines written for that day. If you need to exercise on different days than those listed, then go ahead and do that as long as you get five days of cardio-related physical activity in a seven-day period.

▶ If you don't eat meat, make substitutions appropriately with fish or vegetables.

▶ This week, all shakes and smoothies must be 300 calories or less. Avoid added sugars if possible in those items that you buy in the store.

▶ When cooking or buying your soups, make sure they are 300 calories or less and low in sodium (salt); this means the sodium or Na+ line on the label should say no more than 480 milligrams per serving. Try eating things made with sea salt as it still gives you the flavor, but has less sodium content.

▶ Soups can be consumed with 2 saltine crackers if desired.

▶ The liquid meals must be eaten with either 1 piece of fruit *or* 1 serving of vegetables.

▶ You must consume 1 cup of water before eating a

meal; you must consume 1 cup of water during your meal. You can add lemon or lime to your water and you can drink fizzy water if you desire.

▶ You are allowed to drink coffee, but only 1 small cup per day. Stay away from all of those fancy coffee preparations—lattes, frappucinos—that have a lot of calories. Your coffee should contain no more than 50 calories.

▶ Do not eat the last meal within 90 minutes of going to sleep.

▶ You can eat a 100-calorie snack before going to bed if desired.

▶ Be smart in your snack choices. Avoid chips and doughnuts and candy; you can have them some of the time, but don't eat them often. If you must have something like these items, make it only one of your snacks for the day and use healthier options for the other snacks.

▶ You don't have to eat all of the food on the day's menu if you don't want to, but no skipping meals, no doubling up on meals, and no exceeding the meal guidelines in size and volume.

▶ Condiments like ketchup, mayo, and mustard are allowed, but no more than a teaspoon at each meal. The same goes for soy sauce.

▶ Spices are unlimited.

▶ While fresh fruit is always preferred, canned and frozen fruit are allowed. Just make sure they are water-based and there are no added sugars.

▶ Canned and frozen vegetables are allowed. Please be aware of the sodium content.

▶ As far as beverages are concerned, you are allowed as much water as you like per day. Here are some other beverage guidelines:

No regular soda

1 can of diet soda allowed each day

Flavored waters allowed, but keep them under 60 calories

1 bottle of sports drink allowed per day, but keep under 60 calories

For alcohol, 1 mixed drink allowed twice a week, *or* 3 light beers allowed per week, *or* 3 regular glasses of wine (red or white) allowed per week

SHRED WEEK 1, DAY 1

NOTE: 1 cup of coffee is allowed each day. Please put minimal amounts of sugar and milk in the coffee. Definitely stay away from those coffee concoctions that are full of calories—caramel macchiato, cinnamon dolce latte, caffe latte, etc.

If you choose diet soda as your beverage, you are only allowed to have one 12-ounce can per day maximum. Try to choose beverages that are more nutritious.

Two slices of 100-percent whole-grain or 100-percent whole-wheat bread can be consumed at any point throughout the day at any time; however, *only* 2 slices.

MEAL 1
- 1 piece of fruit
- Choose one of the following:

> 1 small bowl of oatmeal (1½ cups cooked)
>
> 2 egg whites *or* 1 egg-white omelet with diced veggies (made with 2 egg whites max)
>
> 1 small bowl of sugar-free cereal with fat-free, skim, or 1-percent fat milk
>
> 1 container of low-fat or fat-free yogurt

- 1 cup of fresh juice *not* from concentrate (grapefruit, apple, orange juice, tomato, carrot)

SNACK 1

- 100 calories or less

MEAL 2

- Choose one of the following. Your choice must not exceed 300 calories and must not have any added sugars.

  > 1 fruit smoothie
  >
  > 1 protein shake
  >
  > 1 bowl of soup (no potatoes, no cream, no meat). Good choices are vegetable, lentil, chickpea, split pea, black bean, tomato bisque, etc. Be careful of sodium content!

- 1 piece of fruit *or* 1 serving of veggies
- Choose one of the following beverages:

  > One 12-ounce can of diet soda
  >
  > 1 cup of lemonade (freshly squeezed preferred)
  >
  > Unlimited plain water (flat or fizzy)
  >
  > 1 cup of flavored water
  >
  > 1 cup of juice (not from concentrate)
  >
  > 1 cup of unsweetened iced tea or any other type of tea

    1 cup of low-fat, reduced-fat, or fat-free milk, unsweetened soy milk, or unsweetened almond milk

SNACK 2

- 150 calories or less

MEAL 3

- 1 small salad (no bacon bits, no croutons, 3 tablespoons max of fat-free dressing)
- Choose one of the following:

     1 piece of chicken (4–6 ounces, no skin, no frying)

     1 piece of turkey (4–6 ounces, no skin, no frying)

     1 piece of fish (4–6 ounces, no frying)

     You can have 1 slice of cheese if desired.
- 1 serving of veggies
- Choose one of the following beverages. Choose a different beverage from the one you chose in meal 2.

     One 12-ounce can of diet soda

     1 cup of lemonade (freshly squeezed preferred)

     Unlimited plain water (flat or fizzy)

     1 cup of flavored water

     1 cup of juice (not from concentrate)

     1 cup of unsweetened iced tea or any other type of tea

     1 cup of low-fat, reduced-fat, or fat-free milk, unsweetened soy milk, or unsweetened almond milk

MEAL 4

- 3 servings of veggies
- 1 cup of beans (no baked beans)

- Choose one of the following beverages. Try to choose
  a different beverage from what you chose in meals 2
  and 3 if you can. You don't have to, but try.

  One 12-ounce can of diet soda

  1 cup of lemonade (freshly squeezed preferred)

  Unlimited plain water (flat or fizzy)

  1 cup of flavored water

  1 cup of juice (not from concentrate)

  1 cup of unsweetened iced tea or any other type of tea

  1 cup of low-fat, reduced-fat, or fat-free milk, unsweetened soy milk, or unsweetened almond milk

SNACK 3

- 100 calories or less

EXERCISE

- The goal of these exercises is to push yourself to work
  hard in a short period of time. The time listed is how
  much time is expected of you to perform the exercise,
  not how much time you are actually present in the
  gym. A lot of people spend too much time in the gym
  not working out, but talking and posing and doing a
  lot of other things that have nothing to do with the real
  purpose of going to a gym. The clock doesn't start until you are actually moving and the clock stops when
  you stop. To achieve the most results without wasting
  time it's important that you be focused and efficient.
  Do these exercises at moderate levels of intensity. In
  order for these to be effective and have an impact on
  your calorie burn and metabolism, you really need to
  get your heart rate up. You don't have to go to a gym

to do these exercises. You can get a tremendous work-out right in your own house or backyard. Try to choose a workout that's different from the last one you did. Below are some 15-minute interval exercises that you should try. So if the program calls for a 45-minute workout, try 15 minutes on the treadmill, 15 minutes on the bicycle, and 15 minutes on the stair climber. It's up to you how you break it up, but note that changing your routine is typically more advantageous than do-ing the same exercise for the entire workout.

- Amount of exercise today: Minimum 30 minutes. If you want to do more, all the better! Work as hard as you can!

- Choose from this list of cardiovascular exercises. If you need to break up the time into two workout sessions, that's completely acceptable. What's most important is that you actually perform the exercise for the minimum amount of time indicated. The clock only starts when you start exercising, not when you enter the gym.

  Jogging outside
  Walking/running on treadmill
  Elliptical machine
  Stationary or mobile bicycle
  Swimming laps
  Stair climber
  225 jump rope revolutions
  Treadmill walk/run intervals
  Zumba or other type of aerobics
  Spinning class
  Other high-intensity cardio programs
  Rowing machine

SHRED WEEK 1, DAY 2

MEAL 1

- 1 piece of fruit (choose a pear, grapefruit, or apple if possible)
- Choose one of the following:
    - 1 small bowl of oatmeal (1½ cups cooked)
    - 2 egg whites *or* 1 egg-white omelet with diced veggies (made with 2 egg whites max)
    - 1 small bowl of sugar-free cereal with fat-free, skim, or 1-percent fat milk
- 1 piece of 100-percent whole-grain bread or 100-percent whole-wheat toast
- 1 cup of juice *not* from concentrate (grapefruit, apple, orange, carrot, pear, tomato, etc.)

SNACK 1

- 100 calories or less

MEAL 2

- 1 chicken or turkey sandwich on 100-percent whole-wheat or 100-percent whole-grain bread; lettuce, tomato, 1 slice of cheese, and 1 teaspoon of mustard or mayo if desired (You can always substitute a medium salad for a meal. Just remember, only 3 tablespoons of fat-free dressing, no bacon bits, no croutons. Keep it clean.)
- 1 serving of veggies
- Choose one of the following beverages:
    - One 12-ounce can of diet soda

1 cup of lemonade (freshly squeezed preferred)

Unlimited plain water (flat or fizzy)

1 cup of flavored water

1 cup of juice (not from concentrate)

1 cup of unsweetened iced tea or any other type of tea

1 cup of low-fat, reduced-fat, or fat-free milk, un-sweetened soy milk, or unsweetened almond milk

SNACK 2

- 150 calories or less

MEAL 3

- Choose one of the following. Your choice must be 300 calories or less.

    1 fruit smoothie

    1 protein shake

    1 bowl of soup (no potatoes, no cream). Good examples are chicken noodle, vegetable, lentil, chickpea, split pea, black bean, tomato bisque, etc. Be careful of sodium content!

- 1 piece of fruit *or* 1 serving of veggies
- Choose one of the following beverages. Try to choose a different beverage from what you chose in meal 2.

    One 12-ounce can of diet soda

    1 cup of lemonade (freshly squeezed preferred)

    Unlimited plain water (flat or fizzy)

    1 cup of flavored water

    1 cup of juice (not from concentrate)

    1 cup of unsweetened iced tea or any other type of tea

    1 cup of low-fat, reduced-fat, or fat-free milk, un-sweetened soy milk, or unsweetened almond milk

SNACK 3

- 100 calories or less

MEAL 4

- Choose one of the following:

    5-ounce piece of chicken (no skin, no frying)

    5-ounce piece of fish (no frying)

    5-ounce piece of turkey (no skin, no frying)

    (5 ounces is approximately the size of a deck and a half of playing cards.)

- 2 servings of veggies
- Choose one of the following beverages. Try to choose a different beverage from what you chose in meals 2 and 3.

    One 12-ounce can of diet soda

    1 cup of lemonade (freshly squeezed preferred)

    Unlimited plain water (flat or fizzy)

    1 cup of flavored water

    1 cup of juice (not from concentrate)

    1 cup of unsweetened iced tea or any other type of tea

    1 cup of low-fat, reduced-fat, or fat-free milk, unsweetened soy milk, or unsweetened almond milk

EXERCISE

- Amount of exercise today: Minimum 45 minutes. If you want to do more, all the better! Work as hard as you can!
- Choose from this list of cardiovascular exercises. If you need to break up the time into two workout sessions, that's completely acceptable. What's most important is

that you actually perform the exercise for the minimum
amount of time indicated.

Jogging outside

Walking/running on treadmill

Elliptical machine

Stationary or mobile bicycle

Swimming laps

Stair climber

225 jump rope revolutions

Treadmill walk/run intervals

Zumba or other type of aerobics

Spinning class

Other high-intensity cardio programs

Rowing machine

SHRED WEEK 1, DAY 3

MEAL 1

- 1 piece of fruit (choose a pear or grapefruit)
- Choose one of the following:

    1 small bowl of oatmeal (1½ cups cooked)

    2 egg whites *or* an egg-white omelet with diced veggies (made with 2 egg whites max)

    1 small bowl of sugar-free cereal with fat-free, skim, or 1-percent fat milk

    2 pancakes plus 2 strips of bacon (pancakes no bigger than a CD, no more than 1½ tablespoons of syrup, 1 pat of butter; try turkey bacon)

      1 small bowl of Cream of Wheat (1 cup cooked)

      1 6-ounce container of low-fat or fat-free yogurt

- 1 cup of juice *not* from concentrate (grapefruit, apple, orange, carrot, pear, tomato, etc.)

SNACK 1

- 100 calories or less

MEAL 2

- Choose one of the following. Your choice must be 300 calories or less.

  1 fruit smoothie

  1 protein shake

  1 bowl of soup (no potatoes, no cream). Good choices are chicken noodle, vegetable, lentil, chickpea, split pea, black bean, tomato bisque, etc. Be careful of sodium content!

- 1 piece of fruit *or* 1 serving of veggies

- Choose one of the following beverages:

  One 12-ounce can of diet soda

  1 cup of lemonade (freshly squeezed preferred)

  Unlimited plain water (flat or fizzy)

  1 cup of flavored water

  1 cup of juice (not from concentrate)

  1 cup of unsweetened iced tea or any other type of tea

  1 cup of low-fat, reduced-fat, or fat-free milk, unsweetened soy milk, or unsweetened almond milk

SNACK 2

- 150 calories or less

MEAL 3

- 1 chicken or turkey sandwich on 100-percent whole-wheat or 100-percent whole-grain bread; lettuce, tomato, 1 slice of cheese, and 1 teaspoon of mustard or mayo if desired

- 1 small green garden salad (Only 3 tablespoons of fat-free dressing, no bacon bits, no croutons. Keep it clean.)

- Choose one of the following beverages. Try to choose a different beverage from what you chose in meal 2.

    One 12-ounce can of diet soda

    1 cup of lemonade (freshly squeezed preferred)

    Unlimited plain water (flat or fizzy)

    1 cup of flavored water

    1 cup of juice (not from concentrate)

    1 cup of unsweetened iced tea or any other type of tea

    1 cup of low-fat, reduced-fat, or fat-free milk, unsweetened soy milk, or unsweetened almond milk

SNACK 3

- 100 calories or less

MEAL 4

- Choose one of the following:

    5-ounce piece of chicken (no skin, no frying)

    5-ounce piece of fish (no frying)

    5-ounce piece of turkey (no skin, no frying)

    (5 ounces is about the size of a deck and a half of playing cards.)

- ½ cup of cooked brown rice

- 1 serving of veggies
- Choose one of the following beverages. Try to choose a different beverage from what you chose in meals 2 and 3.

    One 12-ounce can of diet soda

    1 cup of lemonade (freshly squeezed preferred)

    Unlimited plain water (flat or fizzy)

    1 cup of flavored water

    1 cup of juice (not from concentrate)

    1 cup of unsweetened iced tea or any other type of tea

    1 cup of low-fat, reduced-fat, or fat-free milk, unsweetened soy milk, or unsweetened almond milk

EXERCISE

- Rest Day. But if you're inspired to do something, by all means go and do it. Every minute of exercise burns more calories and gets you closer to your goal. You might even try playing a sport, which can be a fun way to burn calories without feeling like you're actually working out.

SHRED WEEK 1, DAY 4

MEAL 1

- 1 piece of fruit (choose a pear or grapefruit)
- Choose one of the following. Don't eat the same breakfast every morning if possible.

    1 grilled cheese sandwich on 100-percent whole-grain or 100-percent whole-wheat bread

     1 small bowl of oatmeal (1½ cups cooked)

     2 egg whites *or* an egg-white omelet with diced veggies (made with 2 egg whites max)

     1 small bowl of sugar-free cereal with fat-free, skim, or 1-percent fat milk

     2 pancakes plus 2 strips of bacon (pancakes no bigger than a CD, no more than 1½ tablespoons of syrup, 1 pat of butter; try turkey bacon)

     1 small bowl of Cream of Wheat (1 cup cooked)

- 1 cup of juice *not* from concentrate (grapefruit, apple, orange, carrot, pear, tomato, etc.)

SNACK 1

- 100 calories or less

MEAL 2

- 1 small green garden salad (Only 3 tablespoons of fat-free dressing, no bacon bits, no croutons. Keep it clean.)
- 1 bowl of soup (no potatoes, no cream). Good choices are chicken noodle, vegetable, lentil, chickpea, split pea, black bean, tomato bisque, etc. Be careful of sodium content!
- Choose one of the following beverages:

     One 12-ounce can of diet soda

     1 cup of lemonade (freshly squeezed preferred)

     Unlimited plain water (flat or fizzy)

     1 cup of flavored water

     1 cup of juice (not from concentrate)

     1 cup of unsweetened iced tea or any other type of tea

1 cup of low-fat, reduced-fat, or fat-free milk, unsweetened soy milk, or unsweetened almond milk

SNACK 2

- 150 calories or less

MEAL 3

- 1 fruit smoothie or 1 protein shake (300 calories or less; no added sugar!)
- 1 piece of fruit *or* 1 serving of veggies
- Choose one of the following beverages. Try to choose a different beverage from what you chose in meal 2.

    One 12-ounce can of diet soda

    1 cup of lemonade (freshly squeezed preferred)

    Unlimited plain water (flat or fizzy)

    1 cup of flavored water

    1 cup of juice (not from concentrate)

    1 cup of unsweetened iced tea or any other type of tea

    1 cup of low-fat, reduced-fat, or fat-free milk, unsweetened soy milk, or unsweetened almond milk

SNACK 3

- 100 calories or less

MEAL 4

- Choose one of the following:

    5-ounce piece of lean beef (no frying)

    5-ounce piece of chicken (no skin, no frying)

    5-ounce piece of fish (no frying)

5-ounce piece of turkey (no skin, no frying)

(5 ounces is about the size of a deck and a half of playing cards.)

- 1 serving of veggies
- Half of a baked sweet potato (no whipped cream or other additions; you can add 1 teaspoon of butter)
- Choose one of the following beverages. Try to choose a different beverage from the one you chose in meals 2 and 3.

  One 12-ounce can of diet soda

  1 cup of lemonade (freshly squeezed preferred)

  Unlimited plain water (flat or fizzy)

  1 cup of flavored water

  1 cup of juice (not from concentrate)

  1 cup of unsweetened iced tea or any other type of tea

  1 cup of low-fat, reduced-fat, or fat-free milk, unsweetened soy milk, or unsweetened almond milk

EXERCISE

- Amount of exercise today: Minimum 40 minutes. If you want to do more, all the better! Work as hard as you can!
- Choose from this list of cardiovascular exercises. If you need to break up the time into two workout sessions, that's completely acceptable. What's most important is that you actually perform the exercise for the minimum amount of time indicated. Work hard!

  Jogging outside

  Walking/running on treadmill

Elliptical machine

Stationary or mobile bicycle

Swimming laps

Stair climber

225 jump rope revolutions

Treadmill walk/run intervals

Zumba or other type of aerobics

Spinning class

Other high-intensity cardio programs

Rowing machine

SHRED WEEK 1, DAY 5

MEAL 1

- 1 piece of fruit (choose a different fruit from yesterday's)
- Choose one of the following. Don't eat the same breakfast every morning if possible.

    1 small bowl of oatmeal (1½ cups cooked)

    2 egg whites *or* an egg-white omelet with diced veggies (made with 2 egg whites max)

    1 small bowl of sugar-free cereal with fat-free, skim, or 1-percent fat milk

- 1 cup of juice *not* from concentrate (grapefruit, apple, orange, carrot, pear, tomato, etc.)

SNACK 1

- 100 calories or less

MEAL 2

- 1 fruit smoothie *or* 1 protein shake (300 calories or less; no added sugar!)
- 1 piece of fruit *or* 1 serving of veggies
- Choose one of the following beverages:

    One 12-ounce can of diet soda

    1 cup of lemonade (freshly squeezed preferred)

    Unlimited plain water (flat or fizzy)

    1 cup of flavored water

    1 cup of juice (not from concentrate)

    1 cup of unsweetened iced tea or any other type of tea

    1 cup of low-fat, reduced-fat, or fat-free milk, unsweetened soy milk, or unsweetened almond milk

SNACK 2

- 150 calories or less

MEAL 3

- 1 small green garden salad (Only 1 tablespoon of fat-free dressing, no bacon bits, no croutons. Keep it clean.)
- 1 bowl of soup (no potatoes, no cream). Good choices are chicken noodle, vegetable, lentil, chickpea, split pea, black bean, tomato bisque, etc. Be careful of sodium content!
- Choose one of the following beverages. Try to choose a different beverage from what you chose in meal 2.

    One 12-ounce can of diet soda

    1 cup of lemonade (freshly squeezed preferred)

Unlimited plain water (flat or fizzy)

1 cup of flavored water

1 cup of juice (not from concentrate)

1 cup of unsweetened iced tea or any other type of tea

1 cup of low-fat, reduced-fat, or fat-free milk, unsweetened soy milk, or unsweetened almond milk

SNACK 3

- 100 calories or less

MEAL 4

- Choose one of the following:

    5-ounce piece of chicken (no skin, no frying)

    5-ounce piece of fish (no frying)

    5-ounce piece of turkey (no skin, no frying)

    (5 ounces is about the size of a deck and a half of playing cards.)

- 2 servings of veggies
- Choose one of the following beverages. Try to choose a different beverage from what you chose in meals 2 and 3.

    One 12-ounce can of diet soda

    1 cup of lemonade (freshly squeezed preferred)

    Unlimited plain water (flat or fizzy)

    1 cup of flavored water

    1 cup of juice (not from concentrate)

    1 cup of unsweetened iced tea or any other type of tea

1 cup of low-fat, reduced-fat, or fat-free milk, unsweetened soy milk, or unsweetened almond milk

SNACK 4

- 100 calories or less

EXERCISE

- Amount of exercise today: Minimum 40 minutes. If you want to do more, all the better! Work as hard as you can!
- Choose from this list of cardiovascular exercises. If you need to break up the time into two workout sessions, that's completely acceptable. What's most important is that you actually perform the exercise for the minimum amount of time indicated. Work hard!

  Jogging outside

  Walking/running on treadmill

  Elliptical machine

  Stationary or mobile bicycle

  Swimming laps

  Stair climber

  225 jump rope revolutions

  Treadmill walk/run intervals

  Zumba or other type of aerobics

  Spinning class

  Other high-intensity cardio programs

  Rowing machine

SHRED WEEK 1, DAY 6

MEAL 1

- 1 piece of fruit
- Choose one of the following.

    1 small bowl of oatmeal (1½ cups cooked)

    2 egg whites *or* 1 egg-white omelet with diced veggies (made with 2 egg whites max)

    1 small bowl of sugar-free cereal with fat-free, skim, or 1-percent fat milk

    1 grilled cheese sandwich on 100-percent whole-grain or 100-percent whole-wheat bread

- 1 cup of juice *not* from concentrate (grapefruit, apple, orange, carrot, pear, tomato, etc.)

SNACK 1

- 150 calories or less

MEAL 2

- Choose one of the following. Your choice must be 300 calories or less.

    1 fruit smoothie

    1 protein shake

    1 bowl of soup (no potatoes, no cream). Good choices are chicken noodle, vegetable, lentil, chickpea, split pea, black bean, tomato bisque, etc. Be careful of sodium content!

- 1 piece of fruit *or* 1 serving of veggies
- Choose one of the following beverages:

One 12-ounce can of diet soda

1 cup of lemonade (freshly squeezed preferred)

Unlimited plain water (flat or fizzy)

1 cup of flavored water

1 cup of juice (not from concentrate)

1 cup of unsweetened iced tea or any other type of tea

1 cup of low-fat, reduced-fat, or fat-free milk, unsweetened soy milk, or unsweetened almond milk

SNACK 2

- 100 calories or less

MEAL 3

- Choose one of the following:

    4–6-ounce piece of chicken (no skin, no frying)

    4–6-ounce piece of fish (no frying)

    4–6-ounce piece of turkey (no skin, no frying)

    You can have 1 slice of cheese if desired.

- 1 serving of veggies

- ½ cup of cooked white rice *or* 1 cup of cooked brown rice

- Choose one of the following beverages. Choose a different beverage from what you chose in meal 2.

    One 12-ounce can of diet soda

    1 cup of lemonade (freshly squeezed preferred)

    Unlimited plain water (flat or fizzy)

    1 cup of flavored water

    1 cup of juice (not from concentrate)

    1 cup of unsweetened iced tea or any other type of tea

    1 cup of low-fat, reduced-fat, or fat-free milk, unsweetened soy milk, or unsweetened almond milk

SNACK 3
- 100 calories or less

MEAL 4
- 1 large salad (3 cups of greens; no bacon bits or croutons; 3 tablespoons of fat-free dressing; ¼ cup of shredded cheese allowed)
- 1 cup of beans, chickpeas, lentils, or other legumes (no baked beans)
- Choose one of the following beverages. Choose a different beverage from what you chose in meals 2 and 3.
  One 12-ounce can of diet soda
  1 cup of lemonade (freshly squeezed preferred)
  Unlimited plain water (flat or fizzy)
  1 cup of flavored water
  1 cup of juice (not from concentrate)
  1 cup of unsweetened iced tea or any other type of tea
  1 cup of low-fat, reduced-fat, or fat-free milk, unsweetened soy milk, or unsweetened almond milk

SNACK 4
- Choose one of the following:
  Raw trail mix (½ cup of raw nuts with sunflower or pumpkin seeds and dried fruit)
  2 dates stuffed with almonds (take out the pit and replace with a few almonds)
  ½ cup raisins, raw walnuts, and pinch of sea salt (mix together)
  3 tomato slices and fresh basil drizzled with olive oil

½ cucumber, sliced, sprinkled with a pinch of sea salt and fat-free vinaigrette dressing

1 cup of unsweetened apple sauce

10 cherries mixed with a handful of nuts (cashews, almonds, or walnuts)

8 baby carrots with 2 tablespoons of hummus

Ants on a log (2 celery sticks dabbed with 1 tablespoon of raw nut butter and 1 tablespoon of organic raisins)

1 piece of medium-sized fruit

Small beet salad

1 cup of beet juice

20 almonds

Small fruit cup

8 halves of dried apricots

2 tablespoons of sunflower seeds

4 slices of Melba whole-wheat or whole-grain toast

EXERCISE

- Rest Day. But if you're inspired to do something, by all means go and do it. Every minute of exercise burns more calories and gets you closer to your goal. You might even try playing a sport, which can be a fun way to burn calories without feeling like you're actually working out.

SHRED WEEK 1, DAY 7

MEAL 1

- 1 piece of fruit (choose a pear or grapefruit)
- Choose one of the following:

  1 small bowl of oatmeal (1 ½ cups cooked)

  2 egg whites *or* 1 egg-white omelet with diced veggies (made with 2 egg whites max)

  1 small bowl of sugar-free cereal with fat-free, skim, or 1-percent fat milk

  1 small container of low-fat or fat-free yogurt
- 1 piece of 100-percent whole-grain bread or 100-percent whole-wheat toast
- 1 cup of juice *not* from concentrate (grapefruit, apple, orange, carrot, pear, tomato, etc.)

SNACK 1

- 100 calories or less

MEAL 2

- Choose one of the following. Your choice must be 300 calories or less.

  1 fruit smoothie

  1 protein shake

  1 bowl of soup (no potatoes, no cream). Good choices are chicken noodle, vegetable, lentil, chickpea, split pea, black bean, tomato bisque, etc. Be careful of sodium content!

- 1 piece of fruit *or* 1 serving of veggies
- Choose one of the following beverages:

    One 12-ounce can of diet soda

    1 cup of lemonade (freshly squeezed preferred)

    Unlimited plain water (flat or fizzy)

    1 cup of flavored water

    1 cup of juice (not from concentrate)

    1 cup of unsweetened iced tea or any other type of tea

    1 cup of low-fat, reduced-fat, or fat-free milk, unsweetened soy milk, or unsweetened almond milk

SNACK 2

- 150 calories or less

MEAL 3

- 1 medium salad (no bacon bits, no croutons, 3 tablespoons of fat-free dressing)
- 1 piece of fruit *or* 1 small cup of diced fruit
- Choose one of the following beverages. Choose a different beverage from what you chose in meal 2.

    One 12-ounce can of diet soda

    1 cup of lemonade (freshly squeezed preferred)

    Unlimited plain water (flat or fizzy)

    1 cup of flavored water

    1 cup of juice (not from concentrate)

    1 cup of unsweetened iced tea or any other type of tea

    1 cup of low-fat, reduced-fat, or fat-free milk, unsweetened soy milk, or unsweetened almond milk

SNACK 3

- 100 calories or less

MEAL 4

- Choose one of the following:

    5-ounce piece of chicken (no skin, no frying)

    5-ounce piece of fish (no frying)

    5-ounce piece of turkey (no skin, no frying)

    (5 ounces is about the size of a deck and a half of playing cards.)

- 2 servings of veggies

- Choose one of the following beverages. Choose a different beverage from what you chose in meals 2 and 3.

    One 12-ounce can of diet soda

    1 cup of lemonade (freshly squeezed preferred)

    Unlimited plain water (flat or fizzy)

    1 cup of flavored water

    1 cup of juice (not from concentrate)

    1 cup of unsweetened iced tea or any other type of tea

    1 cup of low-fat, reduced-fat, or fat-free milk, unsweetened soy milk, or unsweetened almond milk

EXERCISE

- Amount of exercise today: Minimum 40 minutes. Complete this workout in two sessions. The first one should be done before 12:00 P.M. the second one done after 2:00 P.M. If you want to do more, all the better! Work as hard as you can!

- Choose from this list of cardiovascular exercises. What's most important is that you actually perform

the exercise for the minimum amount of time indicated.
Work hard!

Jogging outside

Walking/running on treadmill

Elliptical machine

Stationary or mobile bicycle

Swimming laps

Stair climber

225 jump rope revolutions

Treadmill walk/run intervals

Zumba or other type of aerobics

Spinning class

Other high-intensity cardio programs

Rowing machine

CHAPTER 4

Week 2: Challenge

Congratulations on reaching the second leg of your SHRED journey! Remember as we SHRED that it's important to acknowledge and celebrate the small victories just as much as the larger ones. The fact that you've completed your Prime week and you're reading these words right now is a victory. Last week was a chance to work out the kinks. You may not have done all of the required exercises or your food choices may have slipped a little here and there. Not a problem. Now you are ready to Challenge yourself. It's important as you go through this week to remind yourself that progress is only made when you push yourself a little beyond what is familiar or comfortable.

This Challenge week keeps your weight loss rolling right along, but it requires you to be a little more vigilant than you were in the first week. Pay particular attention to the calorie guidelines. This week your shakes, smoothies, and soups must be 250 calories or less. Please pay attention to this and don't get lazy. Don't drink a 300-calorie beverage believing the extra 50 calories won't matter. This is a mistake. Fifty calories here, 20 calories there, add up to be a significant amount at the end of the day. You're working too hard to start getting lazy and cavalier about your calories or choices. When it comes to weight loss, everything counts, whether it's an extra 5 minutes on the treadmill or that extra 25 calories you consume in a snack. Once again, for your convenience, try the snacks and recipes in chapters 9 through 12. These are practical, affordable, and accessible. Use them to your advantage. *Challenge* yourself this week! Believe! Work hard! Have fun!

SHRED WEEK 2 GUIDELINES

▶ Weigh yourself in the morning before starting the program and record it. Don't weigh yourself throughout the week. Your next weigh-in will be the same day the following week in the morning. Weigh yourself in the same manner as you did in the beginning. If you weighed in without wearing clothes initially, then do that again. If you weighed in wearing certain clothes, wear the same clothes for the second weigh-in. Use the same scale both times. *Don't* use a different scale as scales can differ by several pounds.

▶ You must eat something every 3 to 4 hours even if you're not hungry, but *don't* stuff yourself. Eat until you're no longer hungry, but *don't eat until you're full*. If you need less than what's recommended, then great, go ahead and eat less, which is even better. Switching meals is permitted, but try to do it as infrequently as possible. For example, if you know that what's listed for meal 3 is easier to get than what's listed for meal 2, then go ahead and switch. Looking at the day's meals in advance is important as it allows you to best prepare for what's ahead.

▶ Five out of the seven days you must do some type of cardiovascular exercise, commonly called cardio. Pay attention to the guidelines written for that day. If you need to exercise on different days than listed, then go ahead and do that as long as you get five days of cardio-related physical activity in a seven-day period.

▶ If you don't eat meat, make the substitutions appropriately with fish or vegetables.

▶ This week, all shakes and smoothies must be 250 calories or less. This is different from last week, so please pay attention to this change. Avoid added sugars in those items that you buy in the store if possible.

▶ When cooking or buying your soups, make sure they are 250 calories or less and low in sodium (salt); this means the sodium or Na+ line on the label should say no more than 480 milligrams per serving. Try eating things made with sea salt as it still gives you the flavor, but has less sodium content.

▶ Soups can be consumed with 2 saltine crackers if desired.

▶ The liquid meals must be eaten with either 1 piece of fruit *or* 1 serving of vegetables.

▶ You must consume 1 cup of water before eating a meal; you must consume 1 cup of water during your meal. You can add lemon or lime to your water and you can drink fizzy water if you desire.

▶ You are allowed to drink coffee, but only 1 small cup per day. Stay away from all of those fancy coffee preparations that have a lot of calories. Your coffee should contain no more than 50 calories.

▶ Do not eat the last meal within 90 minutes of going to sleep.

▶ You can eat a 100-calorie snack before going to bed if desired.

▶ Be smart in your snack choices. Avoid chips and doughnuts and candy; you can have them some of the time, but don't eat them often. If you must have something like these items, make it only one of your snacks for the day and use healthier options for the other snacks.

▶ You don't have to eat all of the food on the day's menu if you don't want to, but no skipping meals, no doubling up on meals, and no exceeding the meal guidelines in size and volume.

▶ Condiments like ketchup, mayo, and mustard are allowed, but no more than a teaspoon at each meal. The same goes for soy sauce.

▶ Spices are unlimited.

▶ While fresh fruit is always preferred, canned and frozen fruit are allowed. Just make sure they are water based and there are no added sugars.

▶ Canned and frozen vegetables are allowed. Please be aware of the sodium content.

▶ As far as beverages are concerned, you are allowed as much water as you like per day. Here are some other beverage guidelines:

No regular soda
1 can of diet soda allowed each day

Flavored waters allowed, but keep them under 60
calories

1 bottle of a sports drink allowed per day, but keep it
under 60 calories

For alcohol, 1 mixed drink allowed twice a week, *or* 3
light beers allowed per week, *or* 3 regular glasses of
wine (red or white) allowed per week

Timing is critical to the success of this plan. It might
be difficult at first, but plan in advance and do the best
you can. Skipping meals is not advised. Even if you
eat just a small portion, try to eat something on schedule. A sample day's schedule during Challenge might
look something like the grid below, but for each and every day, the order of the meals and snacks is both intended and critical. And on some days, there's a bonus
fourth snack, so follow each day's directions carefully.

8:30 A.M.	10:00 A.M.	11:30 A.M.	1:00 P.M.	3:30 P.M.	7:00 P.M.	8:30 P.M.
Meal 1	Snack 1	Meal 2	Snack 2	Meal 3	Meal 4	Snack 3

SHRED WEEK 2, DAY 1

NOTE: All smoothies, shakes, and soups are 250 calories this week, not
the 300 calories they were last week. If you purchase something that says
it's 300 calories, don't eat/drink all of it, but leave some behind so that
you're not consuming more than the 250 calories. This is *important*!

One cup of coffee is allowed each day. Please put minimal amounts

of sugar and milk in the coffee. Definitely stay away from those coffee concoctions that are full of calories—caramel macchiato, cinnamon dolce
latte, caffe latte, etc.

If you choose the diet soda as your beverage, you are only allowed to
have one 12-ounce can per day maximum. The hope is that you will
choose beverages that are more nutritious.

MEAL 1

- 2 pieces of 100-percent whole-grain or 100-percent
  whole-wheat bread
- 1 piece of fruit
- Choose one of the following:

  1 small bowl of oatmeal (1 ½ cups cooked)

  2 egg whites *or* 1 egg-white omelet with diced veggies (made with 2 egg whites max)

  1 small bowl of sugar-free cereal with fat-free, skim,
  or 1-percent fat milk

- ½ cup of juice *not* from concentrate (grapefruit, apple,
  orange, carrot, pear, tomato, etc.)

SNACK 1

- 100 calories or less

MEAL 2

- Choose one of the following. Your choice must not exceed 250 calories.

  1 fruit smoothie

  1 protein shake

  1 veggie shake (You can use any veggies you want.)

  1 bowl of soup (no potatoes, no cream). Good choices
  are chicken noodle, vegetable, lentil, chickpea, split

pea, black bean, tomato bisque, etc. Be careful of sodium content!

- 1 piece of fruit *or* 1 serving of veggies (the approximate size for 1 serving is the size of your fist)
- Choose one of the following beverages:

  One 12-ounce can of diet soda

  1 cup of lemonade (freshly squeezed preferred)

  Unlimited plain water (flat or fizzy)

  1 cup of flavored water

  1 cup of juice (not from concentrate)

  1 cup of unsweetened iced tea or any other type of tea

  1 cup of low-fat, reduced-fat, or fat-free milk, unsweetened soy milk, or unsweetened almond milk

SNACK 2

- 150 calories or less

MEAL 3

- 1 small green garden salad (Only 3 tablespoons of fat-free dressing, no bacon bits, no croutons. Keep it clean.)
- Choose one of the following:

  4–6-ounce piece of chicken (no skin, no frying)

  4–6-ounce piece of turkey (no skin, no frying)

  4–6-ounce piece of fish (no frying)

  You can have 1 slice of cheese if desired.
- 1 serving of veggies
- Choose one of the following beverages. Choose a different beverage from what you chose in meal 2.

  One 12-ounce can of diet soda

1 cup of lemonade (freshly squeezed preferred)

Unlimited plain water (flat or fizzy)

1 cup of flavored water

1 cup of juice (not from concentrate)

1 cup of unsweetened iced tea or any other type of tea

1 cup of low-fat, reduced-fat, or fat-free milk, unsweetened soy milk, or unsweetened almond milk

MEAL 4

- Choose one of the following. Your choice must not exceed 250 calories. Try to choose something different from what you had in meal 2 if you can. You don't have to, but try.

    1 fruit smoothie

    1 protein shake

    1 veggie shake (You can use any veggies you want.)

    1 bowl of soup (no potatoes, no cream). Good choices are chicken noodle, vegetable, lentil, chickpea, split pea, black bean, tomato bisque, etc. Be careful of sodium content!

- 1 serving of veggies
- Choose one of the following beverages. Try to choose a different beverage from what you chose in meals 2 and 3.

    One 12-ounce can of diet soda

    1 cup of lemonade (freshly squeezed preferred)

    Unlimited plain water (flat or fizzy)

    1 cup of flavored water

    1 cup of juice (not from concentrate)

    1 cup of unsweetened iced tea or any other type of tea

1 cup of low-fat, reduced-fat, or fat-free milk, unsweetened soy milk, or unsweetened almond milk

SNACK 3

- 100 calories or less

EXERCISE

- Amount of exercise today: Minimum 40 minutes. If
  you want to do more, all the better! Work as hard as you
  can!
- Choose from this list of cardiovascular exercises. If you
  need to break up the time into two workout sessions,
  that's completely acceptable. What's most important is
  that you actually perform the exercise for the minimum amount of time indicated.

  Jogging outside

  Walking/running on treadmill

  Elliptical machine

  Stationary or mobile bicycle

  Swimming laps

  Stair climber

  225 jump rope revolutions

  Treadmill walk/run intervals

  Zumba or other type of aerobics

  Spinning class

  Other high-intensity cardio programs

  Rowing machine

SHRED WEEK 2, DAY 2

MEAL 1

- 1 piece of fruit (choose a pear or grapefruit if you can)
- Choose one of the following. Please note that 1 small bowl generally means 1 cup of the cooked food.

  1 small bowl of Cream of Wheat

  1 small bowl of oatmeal (1½ cups cooked)

  2 egg whites *or* 1 egg-white omelet with diced veggies (made with 2 egg whites max)

  1 small bowl of sugar-free cereal with fat-free, skim, or 1-percent fat milk

- 1 piece of 100-percent whole-grain bread or 100-percent whole-wheat toast
- ½ cup of juice *not* from concentrate (grapefruit, apple, orange, carrot, pear, tomato, etc.)

SNACK 1

- 100 calories or less

MEAL 2

- Choose one of the following. Your choice must be 250 calories or less.

  1 fruit smoothie

  1 protein shake

  1 bowl of soup (no potatoes, no cream). Good choices are chicken noodle, vegetable, lentil, chickpea, split pea, black bean, tomato bisque, etc. Be careful of sodium content!

- 1 piece of fruit *or* 1 serving of veggies; if you choose fruit, make it different from what you ate for meal 1.
- Choose one of the following beverages:

    One 12-ounce can of diet soda

    1 cup of lemonade (freshly squeezed preferred)

    Unlimited plain water (flat or fizzy)

    1 cup of flavored water

    1 cup of juice (not from concentrate)

    1 cup of unsweetened iced tea or any other type of tea

    1 cup of low-fat, reduced-fat, or fat-free milk, unsweetened soy milk, or unsweetened almond milk

SNACK 2

- 150 calories or less

MEAL 3

- Choose one of the following. Your choice must be 250 calories or less.

    1 fruit smoothie

    1 protein shake

    1 bowl of soup (no potatoes, no cream). Good choices are chicken noodle, vegetable, lentil, chickpea, split pea, black bean, tomato bisque, etc. Be careful of sodium content!

- 1 piece of fruit *or* 1 serving of veggies
- Choose one of the following beverages. Choose a beverage different from what you chose in meal 2.

    One 12-ounce can of diet soda

    1 cup of lemonade (freshly squeezed preferred)

    Unlimited plain water (flat or fizzy)

1 cup of flavored water

1 cup of juice (not from concentrate)

1 cup of unsweetened iced tea or any other type of tea

1 cup of low-fat, reduced-fat, or fat-free milk, unsweetened soy milk, or unsweetened almond milk

SNACK 3

- 100 calories or less

MEAL 4

- Choose one from the following:

    5-ounce piece of chicken (no skin, no frying)

    5-ounce piece of fish (no frying)

    5-ounce piece of turkey (no skin, no frying)

    (5 ounces is about the size of a deck and a half of playing cards.)

- 2 servings of veggies
- Choose one of the following beverages. Try to choose a different beverage from what you chose in meals 2 and 3.

    One 12-ounce can of diet soda

    1 cup of lemonade (freshly squeezed preferred)

    Unlimited plain water (flat or fizzy)

    1 cup of flavored water

    1 cup of juice (not from concentrate)

    1 cup of unsweetened iced tea or any other type of tea

    1 cup of low-fat, reduced-fat, or fat-free milk, unsweetened soy milk, or unsweetened almond milk

EXERCISE

- Amount of exercise today: Minimum 45 minutes. If you want to do more, all the better! Work as hard as you can!
- Choose from this list of cardiovascular exercises. If you need to break up the time into two workout sessions, that's completely acceptable. What's most important is that you actually perform the exercise for the minimum amount of time indicated.

    Jogging outside

    Walking/running on treadmill

    Elliptical machine

    Stationary or mobile bicycle

    Swimming laps

    Stair climber

    225 jump rope revolutions

    Treadmill walk/run intervals

    Zumba or other type of aerobics

    Spinning class

    Other high-intensity cardio programs

    Rowing machine

SHRED WEEK 2, DAY 3

MEAL 1

- 1 piece of fruit (choose a pear or grapefruit)
- Choose one of the following. Your choice must be 250 calories or less, and no added sugars.

    1 fruit smoothie

    1 protein shake

SNACK 1

- 100 calories or less

MEAL 2

- 1 chicken or turkey sandwich on 100-percent whole-wheat or 100-percent whole-grain bread; lettuce, tomato, 1 slice of cheese, and 1 teaspoon of mustard or mayo if desired
- 1 small green garden salad (Only 3 tablespoons of fat-free dressing, no bacon bits, no croutons. Keep it clean.)
- Choose one of the following beverages:

    One 12-ounce can of diet soda

    1 cup of lemonade (freshly squeezed preferred)

    Unlimited plain water (flat or fizzy)

    1 cup of flavored water

    1 cup of juice (not from concentrate)

    1 cup of unsweetened iced tea or any other type of tea

    1 cup of low-fat, reduced-fat, or fat-free milk, unsweetened soy milk, or unsweetened almond milk

SNACK 2

- 150 calories or less

MEAL 3

- Choose from Group A *or* Group B. *Do not* choose from both:

    Group A—choose one of the following:

    5-ounce piece of chicken (no skin, no frying)

    5-ounce piece of fish (no frying)

    5-ounce piece of turkey (no skin, no frying)

All of the above come with ½ cup of cooked brown rice *and* 1 serving of veggies.

Group B—you can have both items below:

1 serving of lasagna (with or without meat), 4 inches × 2 inches × 1 inch

1 serving of veggies

- Choose one of the following beverages. Choose a different beverage from what you chose in meal 2.

    One 12-ounce can of diet soda

    1 cup of lemonade (freshly squeezed preferred)

    Unlimited plain water (flat or fizzy)

    1 cup of flavored water

    1 cup of juice (not from concentrate)

    1 cup of unsweetened iced tea or any other type of tea

    1 cup of low-fat, reduced-fat, or fat-free milk, unsweetened soy milk, or unsweetened almond milk

SNACK 3

- 100 calories or less

MEAL 4

- Choose one of the following. Your choice must be 250 calories or less. Try to choose something different from what you chose for meal 1. If you can't, it's okay.

    1 fruit smoothie

    1 protein shake

    1 bowl of soup (no potatoes, no cream). Good choices are chicken noodle, vegetable, lentil, chickpea, split pea, black bean, tomato bisque, etc. Be careful of sodium content!

- 1 piece of fruit *or* 1 serving of veggies
- Choose one of the following beverages. Try to choose a different beverage from what you chose in meals 2 and 3.

    One 12-ounce can of diet soda

    1 cup of lemonade (freshly squeezed preferred)

    Unlimited plain water (flat or fizzy)

    1 cup of flavored water

    1 cup of juice (not from concentrate)

    1 cup of unsweetened iced tea or any other type of tea

    1 cup of low-fat, reduced-fat, or fat-free milk, unsweetened soy milk, or unsweetened almond milk

EXERCISE

- Amount of exercise today: Minimum 30 minutes. If you want to do more, all the better! Work as hard as you can!
- Choose from this list of cardiovascular exercises. If you need to break up the time into two workout sessions, that's completely acceptable. What's most important is that you actually perform the exercise for the minimum amount of time indicated. Work hard!

    Jogging outside

    Walking/running on treadmill

    Elliptical machine

    Stationary or mobile bicycle

    Swimming laps

    Stair climber

    225 jump rope revolutions

    Treadmill walk/run intervals

Zumba or other type of aerobics

Spinning class

Other high-intensity cardio programs

Rowing machine

SHRED WEEK 2, DAY 4

MEAL 1

- 1 piece of fruit (choose a pear, grapefruit, or orange if possible)
- Choose one from the following. Don't eat the same breakfast every morning if possible.

    1 grilled cheese sandwich on 100-percent whole-grain or 100-percent whole-wheat bread

    1 small bowl of oatmeal (1½ cups cooked)

    2 egg whites *or* an egg-white omelet with diced veggies (made with 2 egg whites max)

    1 small bowl of sugar-free cereal with fat-free, skim, or 1-percent fat milk

    2 pancakes plus 2 strips of bacon (no more than 5 inches in diameter, no more than 1½ tablespoons of syrup, 1 pat of butter; try turkey bacon)

    1 small bowl of Cream of Wheat

- 1 cup of juice *not* from concentrate (grapefruit, apple, orange, carrot, pear, tomato, etc.)

SNACK 1

- 100 calories or less

MEAL 2

- 1 fruit smoothie *or* 1 protein shake (250 calories or less; no added sugar)
- 1 piece of fruit *or* 1 serving of veggies
- Choose one of the following beverages:

    One 12-ounce can of diet soda

    1 cup of lemonade (freshly squeezed preferred)

    Unlimited plain water (flat or fizzy)

    1 cup of flavored water

    1 cup of juice (not from concentrate)

    1 cup of unsweetened iced tea or any other type of tea

    1 cup of low-fat, reduced-fat, or fat-free milk, unsweetened soy milk, or unsweetened almond milk

SNACK 2

- 150 calories or less

MEAL 3

- Choose from one of the following. Your choice must be 250 calories or less, and no sugar added.

    1 fruit smoothie

    1 protein shake

    1 bowl of soup (no potatoes, no cream). Good choices are chicken noodle, vegetable, lentil, chickpea, split pea, black bean, tomato bisque, etc. Be careful of sodium content!
- 1 piece of fruit *or* 1 serving of veggies
- Choose one of the following beverages. Choose a different beverage from what you chose in meal 2.

One 12-ounce can of diet soda

1 cup of lemonade (freshly squeezed preferred)

Unlimited plain water (flat or fizzy)

1 cup of flavored water

1 cup of juice (not from concentrate)

1 cup of unsweetened iced tea or any other type of tea

1 cup of low-fat, reduced-fat, or fat-free milk, unsweetened soy milk, or unsweetened almond milk

SNACK 3
- 100 calories or less

MEAL 4
- Choose one from the following.

    5-ounce piece of lean beef (no frying)

    5-ounce piece of chicken (no skin, no frying)

    5-ounce piece of fish (no frying)

    5-ounce piece of turkey (no skin, no frying)

    1 cup of spaghetti and meatballs

    (5 ounces is about the size of a deck and a half of playing cards.)
- 1 serving of veggies
- Half of a baked sweet potato (no whipped cream or other additions; you can add 1 teaspoon of butter)
- Choose one of the following beverages. Try to choose a different beverage from what you chose in meals 2 and 3.

    One 12-ounce can of diet soda

    1 cup of lemonade (freshly squeezed preferred)

    Unlimited plain water (flat or fizzy)

1 cup of flavored water

1 cup of juice (not from concentrate)

1 cup of unsweetened iced tea or any other type of tea

1 cup of low-fat, reduced-fat or fat-free milk, unsweetened soy milk, or unsweetened almond milk

EXERCISE

- Rest Day. But if you're inspired to do something, by all means go and do it. Every minute of exercise burns more calories and gets you closer to your goal. You might even try playing a sport, which can be a fun way to burn calories without feeling like you're actually working out.

SHRED WEEK 2, DAY 5

MEAL 1

- Choose one of the following. Your choice must be 250 calories or less.

    1 fruit smoothie

    1 protein shake

    1 veggie shake

- 1 cup of low-fat or fat-free yogurt
- ½ cup of juice *not* from concentrate (grapefruit, apple, orange, carrot, pear, tomato, etc.)

SNACK 1

- 150 calories or less

MEAL 2

- Choose one of the following. Your choice must be less than 250 calories and no sugar added. Try to choose something different from what you chose in meal 1.

    1 fruit smoothie

    1 protein shake

    1 veggie shake

- 1 piece of fruit *or* 1 serving of veggies
- Choose one of the following beverages:

    One 12-ounce can of diet soda

    1 cup of lemonade (freshly squeezed preferred)

    Unlimited plain water (flat or fizzy)

    1 cup of flavored water

    1 cup of juice (not from concentrate)

    1 cup of unsweetened iced tea or any other type of tea

    1 cup of low-fat, reduced-fat, or fat-free milk, unsweetened soy milk, or unsweetened almond milk

SNACK 2

- 150 calories or less

MEAL 3

- 1 medium green garden salad (Only 3 tablespoons of fat-free dressing, no bacon bits, no croutons. Keep it clean.)
- 1 cup of soup less than 250 calories (no potatoes, no cream). Good choices are chicken noodle, vegetable, lentil, chickpea, split pea, black bean, tomato bisque, etc. Be careful of sodium content!

- Choose one of the following beverages. Choose a different beverage from what you chose in meal 2.

    One 12-ounce can of diet soda

    1 cup of lemonade (freshly squeezed preferred)

    Unlimited plain water (flat or fizzy)

    1 cup of flavored water

    1 cup of juice (not from concentrate)

    1 cup of unsweetened iced tea or any other type of tea

    1 cup of low-fat, reduced-fat, or fat-free milk, unsweetened soy milk, or unsweetened almond milk

SNACK 3

- 150 calories or less

MEAL 4

- Choose one from the following:

    5-ounce piece of chicken (no skin, no frying)

    5-ounce piece of fish (no frying)

    5-ounce piece of turkey (no skin, no frying)

    (5 ounces is about the size of a deck and a half of playing cards.)

- 2 servings of veggies

- Choose one of the following beverages. Try to choose a different beverage from what you chose in meals 2 and 3.

    One 12-ounce can of diet soda

    1 cup of lemonade (freshly squeezed preferred)

    Unlimited plain water (flat or fizzy)

    1 cup of flavored water

1 cup of juice (not from concentrate)

1 cup of unsweetened iced tea or any other type of tea

1 cup of low-fat, reduced-fat, or fat-free milk, unsweetened soy milk, or unsweetened almond milk

SNACK 4

- 100 calories or less

EXERCISE

- Amount of exercise today: Minimum 40 minutes. If you want to do more, all the better! Work as hard as you can!
- Choose from this list of cardiovascular exercises. If you need to break up the time into two workout sessions, that's completely acceptable. What's most important is that you actually perform the exercise for the minimum amount of time indicated. Work hard!

  Jogging outside

  Walking/running on treadmill

  Elliptical machine

  Stationary or mobile bicycle

  Swimming laps

  Stair climber

  225 jump rope revolutions

  Treadmill walk/run intervals

  Zumba or other type of aerobics

  Spinning class

  Other high-intensity cardio programs

  Rowing machine

SHRED WEEK 2, DAY 6

MEAL 1

- 1 piece of fruit
- Choose one of the following:

  1 small bowl of oatmeal (1½ cups cooked)

  2 egg whites *or* 1 egg-white omelet with diced veggies (made with 2 egg whites max)

  1 small bowl of sugar-free cereal with fat-free, skim, or 1-percent fat milk

  1 grilled cheese on 100-percent whole-grain or 100-percent whole-wheat bread

- 1 cup of juice *not* from concentrate (grapefruit, apple, orange, carrot, pear, tomato, etc.)

SNACK 1

- 150 calories or less

MEAL 2

- Choose one from the following. Your choice must be 250 calories or less.

  1 fruit smoothie

  1 protein shake

  1 bowl of soup (no potatoes, no cream, no meat). Good choices are vegetable, lentil, chickpea, split pea, black bean, tomato bisque, etc. Be careful of sodium content!

- 1 piece of fruit *or* 1 serving of veggies

- Choose one of the following beverages:

     One 12-ounce can of diet soda

     1 cup of lemonade (freshly squeezed preferred)

     Unlimited plain water (flat or fizzy)

     1 cup of flavored water

     1 cup of juice (not from concentrate)

     1 cup of unsweetened iced tea or any other type of tea

     1 cup of low-fat, reduced-fat, or fat-free milk, unsweetened soy milk, or unsweetened almond milk

SNACK 2

- 100 calories or less

MEAL 3

- Choose one of the following. Your choice must be 250 calories or less. Try to choose something different from what you chose in meal 2.

     1 fruit smoothie

     1 protein shake

     1 bowl of soup (no potatoes, no cream, no meat). Good choices are vegetable, lentil, chickpea, split pea, black bean, tomato bisque, etc. Be careful of sodium content!

- 1 piece of fruit *or* 1 serving of veggies
- Choose one of the following beverages. Choose a different beverage from what you chose in meal 2.

     One 12-ounce can of diet soda

     1 cup of lemonade (freshly squeezed preferred)

     Unlimited plain water (flat or fizzy)

     1 cup of flavored water

1 cup of juice (not from concentrate)

1 cup of unsweetened iced tea or any other type of tea

1 cup of low-fat, reduced-fat, or fat-free milk, unsweetened soy milk, or unsweetened almond milk

SNACK 3

- 100 calories or less

MEAL 4

- 1 large salad (3 cups of greens; no bacon bits or croutons; 3 tablespoons fat-free dressing allowed; ¼ cup of shredded cheese allowed)
- 1 cup of beans (no baked beans)

SNACK 4

- Choose one of the following:

    20 almonds

    2 rice cakes with 1 teaspoon of peanut butter

    Small fruit cup

    8 halves of dried apricots

    2 tablespoons of sunflower seeds

    4 slices of Melba whole-wheat or whole-grain toast

EXERCISE

- Amount of exercise today: Minimum 30 minutes. If you want to do more, all the better! Work as hard as you can!
- Choose from this list of cardiovascular exercises. If you need to break up the time into two workout sessions,

that's completely acceptable. What's most important is that you actually perform the exercise for the minimum amount of time indicated. Work hard!

Jogging outside

Walking/running on treadmill

Elliptical machine

Stationary or mobile bicycle

Swimming laps

Stair climber

225 jump rope revolutions

Treadmill walk/run intervals

Zumba or other type of aerobics

Spinning class

Other high-intensity cardio programs

Rowing machine

SHRED WEEK 2, DAY 7

MEAL 1

- Choose one of the following. Your choice must be 250 calories or less.

    1 fruit smoothie

    1 protein shake

    1 veggie shake

- 1 piece of fruit

SNACK 1

- 100 calories or less

MEAL 2

- 1 chicken or turkey sandwich on 100-percent whole-wheat or 100-percent whole-grain bread; lettuce, tomato, 1 slice of cheese, and 1 teaspoon of mustard or mayo if desired
- 1 small green garden salad (Only 3 tablespoons of fat-free dressing, no bacon bits, no croutons. Keep it clean.)
- Choose one of the following beverages:

  One 12-ounce can of diet soda

  1 cup of lemonade (freshly squeezed preferred)

  Unlimited plain water (flat or fizzy)

  1 cup of flavored water

  1 cup of juice (not from concentrate)

  1 cup of unsweetened iced tea or any other type of tea

  1 cup of low-fat, reduced-fat, or fat-free milk, unsweetened soy milk, or unsweetened almond milk

SNACK 2

- 150 calories or less

MEAL 3

- Choose one of the following. Your choice must be 250 calories or less.

  1 fruit smoothie

  1 protein shake

  1 veggie shake

  1 bowl of soup (no potatoes, no cream). Good choices are chicken noodle, vegetable, lentil, chickpea, split pea, black bean, tomato bisque, etc. Be careful of sodium content!

- 1 piece of fruit *or* 1 serving of veggies
- Choose one of the following beverages. Choose a beverage different from the one you chose in meal 2.

    One 12-ounce can of diet soda

    1 cup of lemonade (freshly squeezed preferred)

    Unlimited plain water (flat or fizzy)

    1 cup of flavored water

    1 cup of juice (not from concentrate)

    1 cup of unsweetened iced tea or any other type of tea

    1 cup of low-fat, reduced-fat, or fat-free milk, unsweetened soy milk, or unsweetened almond milk

SNACK 3

- 100 calories or less

MEAL 4

- Choose one of the following:

    5-ounce piece of chicken (no skin, no frying)

    5-ounce piece of fish (no frying)

    5-ounce piece of turkey (no skin, no frying)

    (5 ounces is about the size of a deck and a half of playing cards.)

- 1 serving of veggies
- ½ cup of cooked brown *or* white rice
- Choose one of the following beverages. Choose a different beverage from what you chose in meals 2 and 3.

    One 12-ounce can of diet soda

    1 cup of lemonade (freshly squeezed preferred)

    Unlimited plain water (flat or fizzy)

    1 cup of flavored water

1 cup of juice (not from concentrate)

1 cup of unsweetened iced tea or any other type of tea

1 cup of low-fat, reduced-fat, or fat-free milk, unsweetened soy milk, or unsweetened almond milk

EXERCISE

- Rest Day. But if you're inspired to do something, by all means go and do it. Every minute of exercise burns more calories and gets you closer to your goal. You might even try playing a sport, which can be a fun way to burn calories without feeling like you're actually working out.

CHAPTER 5

Week 3: Transformation

Awesome! You have reached the third week as a SHREDDER. You have now demonstrated two things: First, you've shown that you have the tenacity to keep going and make it to this point; second, you've shown that you are taking this plan and reaching your goals seriously. This is the point where many start having doubts and are vulnerable to the temptation to quit. This week requires your mental fortitude more than any other week of the program. You are now going to truly undergo a Transformation.

Week 3 is designed to be the toughest week of the program. This is important, because your body has lost some weight and is starting to adapt to the eating and exercise changes, but what you don't know is that it's fighting with all its might to hold on to the fat and prevent you from losing more weight. This is otherwise known as a plateau. It's important to understand that plateaus are a good and bad thing. They are good because they are your body's confirmation that you are winning the battle and SHREDDING fat. The body's natural desire is not to shed fat, rather to hold on to it and conserve energy. The bad news is that a plateau means your weight loss has stopped or slowed and now you need to find a way to get rolling again. This is what

Transformation is all about. This week is designed for you to keep winning the battle.

The stakes are extremely high now, which means total commitment is needed to succeed. There is a new calorie guideline. Last week you could have 250 calories in your shakes, smoothies, and soups. This week that number drops to 200. This is a strategic decision, so pay close attention to this new number. Your exercise is more critical than ever as your body is trying to conserve energy and hold on to that fat. Get all of your exercise in and push yourself during some workouts for a little bonus. You have already demonstrated your ability to work hard and get the job done—so don't stop now. This is your week to *Transform*! Believe! Work hard! Have fun!

SHRED WEEK 3 GUIDELINES

▶ Weigh yourself in the morning before starting the program and record it. Don't weigh yourself throughout the week. Your next weigh-in will be the same day the following week in the morning. Weigh yourself in the same manner as you did in the beginning. If you weighed in without wearing clothes initially, then do that again. If you weighed in wearing certain clothes, wear the same clothes for the second weigh-in. Use the same scale both times. *Don't* use a different scale as scales can differ by several pounds.

▶ You must eat something every 3 to 4 hours even if you're not hungry, but *don't* stuff yourself. Eat until you're no longer hungry, but *don't eat until you're full*. If you need less than what's recommended, then great, go ahead and eat less, which is even better. Switching meals is permitted, but try to switch as infrequently as possible. For example, if you know that what's listed for meal 3 is easier to get than what's listed for meal 2, then go ahead and switch them. Looking at the day's meals in advance is important as it allows you to best prepare for what's ahead.

▶ Five of the seven days you must do some type of cardiovascular exercise, commonly called cardio. Pay attention to the guidelines written for that day. If you need to exercise on different days than listed, then go ahead and do that as long as you get five days of cardio-related physical activity in a seven-day period.

▶ If you don't eat meat, make the substitutions appropriately with fish or vegetables.

▶ This week all shakes and smoothies must be 200 calories or less. This is different from last week, so please pay attention to this change. Avoid added sugars in those items that you buy in the store if possible.

▶ When cooking or buying your soups, make sure they are 200 calories or less and low in sodium (salt); this means the sodium or Na+ line on the label should say no more than 480 milligrams per serving. Try eating things made with sea salt as it still gives you the flavor but has less sodium content.

▶ Read the label of the products carefully to make sure you're only consuming the amount that corresponds to the calorie limit. Here is an example of a scenario you might find. Let's take a large can of soup whose nutritional label might say something like this:

Calories per serving: 100
Servings: 3
Serving size: 1 cup

This means the can contains 3 servings and each serving has 100 calories. So if you were to eat the entire can, you would be consuming 300 calories. This is something you must not do this week. So to make sure you don't go over the 200 calories, you can consume 2 cups of the soup. Here is the simple math.

1 SERVING	+	1 SERVING	=	2 SERVINGS
100 cal	+	100 cal	=	200 cals

1 CUP	+	1 CUP	=	2 CUPS
So, 200 cals	=	2 servings	=	2 cups

▶ Remember, if you are uncertain, always err on the side of caution and consume less than the 200 calories rather than more. Success this particular week will be optimized by how closely you follow the instructions regarding quantity, timing, and food selections. Work hard this week. It will be your toughest, but very doable.

▶ Soups can be consumed with the 2 saltine crackers if desired.

▶ The liquid meals must be eaten with either 1 piece of fruit or 1 serving of vegetables.

▶ You must consume 1 cup of water before eating a meal; you must consume 1 cup of water during your meal. You can add lemon or lime to your water and you can drink fizzy water if you desire.

▶ You are allowed to drink coffee, but only 1 small cup per day. Stay away from all of those fancy coffee preparations that have a lot of calories. Your coffee should contain no more than 50 calories.

▶ Do not eat the last meal within 90 minutes of going to sleep.

▶ You can eat a 100-calorie snack before going to bed if desired.

▶ Be smart in your snack choices. Avoid chips and doughnuts and candy; you can have them some of the time, but don't eat them often. If you must have something like these items, make it only one of your snacks for the day and use healthier options for the other snacks.

▶ You don't have to eat all of the food on the day's menu if you don't want to, but no skipping meals, no doubling up on meals, and no exceeding the meal guidelines in size and volume.

▶ Condiments such as ketchup, mayo, and mustard are allowed, but no more than a teaspoon at each meal. The same goes for soy sauce.

▶ Spices are unlimited.

▶ While fresh fruit is always preferred, canned and frozen fruit are allowed. Just make sure they are water-based and there are no added sugars.

▶ Canned and frozen vegetables are allowed. Please be aware of the sodium content.

▶ As far as beverages are concerned, you are allowed as much water as you like per day. Here are some other beverage guidelines:

No regular soda
1 can of diet soda allowed each day
Flavored waters allowed, but keep them under 60 calories
1 bottle of sports drink allowed per day, but keep it under 60 calories
For alcohol, 1 mixed drink allowed twice a week, *or* 3 light beers allowed per week, *or* 3 regular glasses of wine (red or white) allowed per week

Timing is critical to the success of this plan. It might be difficult at first, but plan in advance and do the best you can. Skipping meals is not advised. Even if you eat just a small portion, try to eat something on schedule. A sample day's schedule during Transformation might look something like the grid below, but for each and every day, the order of the meals and snacks is both intended and critical. And on some days, there's a bonus fourth snack, so follow each day's directions carefully.

8:30 A.M.	10:00 A.M.	11:30 A.M.	1:00 P.M.	3:30 P.M.	7:00 P.M.	8:30 P.M.
Meal 1	Snack 1	Meal 2	Snack 2	Meal 3	Meal 4	Snack 3

SHRED WEEK 3, DAY 1

NOTE: All smoothies, shakes, and soups are 200 calories this week, not the 250 calories they were last week. If you purchase something that is 250 or more calories, don't eat/drink all of it, but leave some behind so that you're not consuming more than the 200 calories. This is *important*!

One cup of coffee is allowed each day. Please put minimal amounts of sugar and milk in the coffee. Definitely stay away from those coffee concoctions that are full of calories—caramel macchiato, cinnamon dolce latte, caffe latte, etc.

If you choose diet soda as your beverage, you are only allowed to have one 12-ounce can per day maximum. The hope is that you will choose beverages that are more nutritious.

MEAL 1

- 1 cup of lemon water. Pour 8 ounces of water, either hot or cold. Squeeze the juice from half a lemon directly into the water. If you like, add ½ teaspoon of sugar. Mix well and drink.
- 1 piece of fruit. This can be 1 banana, 1 apple, 1 pear, etc. It can also be ½ cup of raspberries, blueberries, blackberries, or strawberries.
- Choose only one of the following:

    1 small bowl of oatmeal (1 ½ cups cooked)

    2 egg whites *or* 1 egg-white omelet with diced veggies (made with 2 egg whites max)

    1 small bowl of sugar-free cereal with fat-free, skim, or 1-percent fat milk
- ½ cup of fresh grapefruit, apple, or orange juice

SNACK 1

- 100 calories or less

MEAL 2

- Choose one of the following. Your choice must not exceed 200 calories.

  1 milk shake (must be made with low-fat or skim milk)

  1 fruit smoothie

  1 protein shake

  1 veggie shake (You can use any veggies you want.)

- 1 piece of fruit *or* 1 serving of veggies. Make sure the fruit chosen is different from what you ate for the first meal.

- Choose one of the following beverages:

  One 12-ounce can of diet soda

  1 cup of lemonade (freshly squeezed preferred)

  Unlimited plain water (flat or fizzy)

  1 cup of flavored water

  1 cup of juice (not from concentrate)

  1 cup of unsweetened iced tea or any other type of tea

  1 cup of low-fat, reduced-fat, or fat-free milk, unsweetened soy milk, or unsweetened almond milk

SNACK 2

- 150 calories or less

MEAL 3

- Choose one of the following. Your choice must not exceed 200 calories. Try to choose something different

from what you had in meal 2 if you can. You don't
have to, but try.

1 milk shake

1 fruit smoothie

1 protein shake

1 veggie shake (You can use any veggies you want.)

1 bowl of soup (no potatoes, no cream). Good choices
are chicken noodle, vegetable, lentil, chickpea, split
pea, black bean, tomato bisque, etc. Be careful of sodium content!

- Choose one of the following beverages. Choose a different beverage from what you chose for meal 2.

One 12-ounce can of diet soda

1 cup of lemonade (freshly squeezed preferred)

Unlimited plain water (flat or fizzy)

1 cup of flavored water

1 cup of juice (not from concentrate)

1 cup of unsweetened iced tea or any other type of
tea

1 cup of low-fat, reduced-fat, or fat-free milk, unsweetened soy milk, or unsweetened almond milk

MEAL 4

- Choose one of the following. Your choice must not exceed 200 calories. Try to choose something different
from what you chose in meals 2 and 3 if you can. You
don't have to, but try.

1 milk shake

1 fruit smoothie

1 protein shake

1 veggie shake (You can use any veggies you want.)

- 1 bowl of soup (no potatoes, no cream). Good choices are chicken noodle, vegetable, lentil, chickpea, split pea, black bean, tomato bisque, etc. Be careful of sodium content!
- 1 piece of fruit *or* 1 serving of veggies
- Choose one of the following beverages. Choose a different beverage from what you chose in meals 2 and 3.

    One 12-ounce can of diet soda

    1 cup of lemonade (freshly squeezed preferred)

    Unlimited plain water (flat or fizzy)

    1 cup of flavored water

    1 cup of juice (not from concentrate)

    1 cup of unsweetened iced tea or any other type of tea

    1 cup of low-fat, reduced-fat, or fat-free milk, unsweetened soy milk, or unsweetened almond milk

SNACK 3

- 100 calories or less

EXERCISE

- Amount of exercise today: Minimum 40 minutes. If you want to do more, all the better! Work as hard as you can!
- Choose from this list of cardiovascular exercises. If you need to break up the time into two workout sessions, that's completely acceptable. What's most important is that you actually perform the exercise for the minimum amount of time indicated. Work hard!

    Jogging outside

    Walking/running on treadmill

    Elliptical machine

Stationary or mobile bicycle

Swimming laps

Stair climber

225 jump rope revolutions

Treadmill walk/run intervals

Zumba or other type of aerobics

Spinning class

Other high-intensity cardio programs

Rowing machine

SHRED WEEK 3, DAY 2

MEAL 1

- 1 cup of lemon water. Pour 8 ounces of water, either hot
  or cold. Squeeze the juice from half a lemon directly
  into the water. If you prefer, add ½ teaspoon of sugar.
  Mix well and drink.
- Choose one of the following. Your choice must be 200
  calories or less.

    1 fruit smoothie

    1 protein shake

SNACK 1

- 100 calories or less

MEAL 2

- Choose one of the following. Your choice must be 200
  calories or less. Choose something different from what
  you chose for meal 1.

    1 fruit smoothie

    1 protein shake

- 1 piece of fruit *or* 1 serving of green leafy veggies
- Choose one of the following beverages:

    One 12-ounce can of diet soda

    1 cup of lemonade (freshly squeezed preferred)

    Unlimited plain water (flat or fizzy)

    1 cup of flavored water

    1 cup of juice (not from concentrate)

    1 cup of unsweetened iced tea or any other type of tea

    1 cup of low-fat, reduced-fat, or fat-free milk, unsweetened soy milk, or unsweetened almond milk

SNACK 2

- 150 calories or less

MEAL 3

- Choose one of the following. Your choice must be 200 calories or less. Make your selection different from what you did for meal 2.

    1 fruit smoothie

    1 protein shake

    1 bowl of soup (no potatoes, no cream). Good choices are chicken noodle, vegetable, lentil, chickpea, split pea, black bean, tomato bisque, etc. Be careful of sodium content!

- 1 piece of fruit *or* 1 serving of leafy green veggies
- Choose one of the following beverages. Choose a different beverage from what you chose in meal 2.

    One 12-ounce can of diet soda

    1 cup of lemonade (freshly squeezed preferred)

Unlimited plain water (flat or fizzy)

1 cup of flavored water

1 cup of juice (not from concentrate)

1 cup of unsweetened iced tea or any other type of tea

1 cup of low-fat, reduced-fat, or fat-free milk, un-sweetened soy milk, or unsweetened almond milk

SNACK 3

- 100 calories or less

MEAL 4

- Choose one of the following. Your choice must be 200 calories or less. Choose something different from what you did for meal 3.

    1 fruit smoothie

    1 protein shake

    1 bowl of soup (no potatoes, no cream). Good choices are chicken noodle, vegetable, lentil, chickpea, split pea, black bean, tomato bisque, etc. Be careful of sodium content!

- 1 serving of veggies
- Choose one of the following beverages. Choose a beverage different from what you chose for meals 2 and 3.

    One 12-ounce can of diet soda

    1 cup of lemonade (freshly squeezed preferred)

    Unlimited plain water (flat or fizzy)

    1 cup of flavored water

    1 cup of juice (not from concentrate)

    1 cup of unsweetened iced tea or any other type of tea

    1 cup of low-fat, reduced-fat, or fat-free milk, un-sweetened soy milk, or unsweetened almond milk

EXERCISE

- Amount of exercise today: Minimum 45 minutes. If you want to do more, all the better! Work as hard as you can!
- Choose from this list of cardiovascular exercises. If you need to break up the time into two workout sessions, that's completely acceptable. What's most important is that you actually perform the exercise for the minimum amount of time indicated. Work hard!

  Jogging outside

  Walking/running on treadmill

  Elliptical machine

  Stationary or mobile bicycle

  Swimming laps

  Stair climber

  225 jump rope revolutions

  Treadmill walk/run intervals

  Zumba or other type of aerobics

  Spinning class

  Other high-intensity cardio programs

  Rowing machine

SHRED WEEK 3, DAY 3

MEAL 1

- 1 cup of lemon water. Pour 8 ounces of water, either hot or cold. Squeeze the juice of half a lemon directly into the water. If you prefer, add ½ teaspoon of sugar. Mix well and drink.

- 1 piece of fruit. This can be 1 banana, 1 apple, 1 pear, etc. It can also be ½ cup of raspberries, blueberries, blackberries, or strawberries.
- Choose one of the following. Your portion should be about 1 cup cooked.

    1 small bowl of oatmeal

    1 small bowl of Cream of Wheat

    1 small bowl of grits

SNACK 1

- 100 calories or less

MEAL 2

- Choose one of the following. Your choice must not exceed 200 calories.

    1 milk shake

    1 fruit smoothie

    1 protein shake

    1 veggie shake (You can use any veggies you want.)

- 1 piece of fruit
- Choose one of the following beverages:

    One 12-ounce can of diet soda

    1 cup of lemonade (freshly squeezed preferred)

    Unlimited plain water (flat or fizzy)

    1 cup of flavored water

    1 cup of juice (not from concentrate)

    1 cup of unsweetened iced tea or any other type of tea

    1 cup of low-fat, reduced-fat, or fat-free milk, unsweetened soy milk, or unsweetened almond milk

SNACK 2

- 150 calories or less

MEAL 3

- Choose one of the following. Your choice must not exceed 200 calories. Try to choose something different from what you had in meal 2 if you can. You don't have to, but try.

  1 milk shake

  1 fruit smoothie

  1 protein shake

  1 veggie shake (You can use any veggies you want.)

  1 bowl of soup (no potatoes, no cream) Good choices are chicken noodle, vegetable, lentil, chickpea, split pea, black bean, tomato bisque, etc. Be careful of sodium content!

- Choose one of the following beverages:

  One 12-ounce can of diet soda

  1 cup of lemonade (freshly squeezed preferred)

  Unlimited plain water (flat or fizzy)

  1 cup of flavored water

  1 cup of juice (not from concentrate)

  1 cup of unsweetened iced tea or any other type of tea

  1 cup of low-fat, reduced-fat, or fat-free milk, unsweetened soy milk, or unsweetened almond milk

SNACK 3

- 100 calories or less

MEAL 4

- Choose one of the following. Your choice must not exceed 200 calories. Try to choose something different from what you had in meal 3 if you can. You don't have to, but try.

  1 milk shake

  1 fruit smoothie

  1 protein shake

  1 veggie shake (You can use any veggies you want.)

  1 bowl of soup (no potatoes, no cream). Good choices are chicken noodle, vegetable, lentil, chickpea, split pea, black bean, tomato bisque, etc. Be careful of sodium content!

- 1 serving of veggies (Remember, the serving size is the size of your fist!)

- Choose one of the following beverages:

  One 12-ounce can of diet soda

  1 cup of lemonade (freshly squeezed preferred)

  Unlimited plain water (flat or fizzy)

  1 cup of flavored water

  1 cup of juice (not from concentrate)

  1 cup of unsweetened iced tea or any other type of tea

  1 cup of low-fat, reduced-fat, or fat-free milk, unsweetened soy milk, or unsweetened almond milk

EXERCISE

- Amount of exercise today: Minimum 30 minutes. If you want to do more, all the better! Work as hard as you can!

- Choose from this list of cardiovascular exercises. If you need to break up the time into two workout sessions, that's completely acceptable. What's most important is that you actually perform the exercise for the minimum amount of time indicated. Work hard!

  Jogging outside

  Walking/running on treadmill

  Elliptical machine

  Stationary or mobile bicycle

  Swimming laps

  Stair climber

  225 jump rope revolutions

  Treadmill walk/run intervals

  Zumba or other type of aerobics

  Spinning class

  Other high-intensity cardio programs

  Rowing machine

SHRED WEEK 3, DAY 4

MEAL 1

- 1 cup of lemon water. Pour 8 ounces of water, either hot or cold. Squeeze the juice from half a lemon directly into the water. If you prefer, add ½ teaspoon of sugar. Mix well and drink.
- 1 cup of raspberries, sliced strawberries, blueberries, or blackberries
- Choose one of the following. Your choice must be 200 calories or less and no sugar added.

    1 fruit smoothie

    1 protein shake

SNACK 1

- 100 calories or less

MEAL 2

- Choose one of the following. Your choice must be 200 calories or less and no sugar added. Try to choose something different from meal 1.

    1 fruit smoothie

    1 protein shake

    1 veggie shake

- 1 piece of fruit *or* 1 serving of veggies
- Choose one of the following beverages:

    One 12-ounce can of diet soda

    1 cup of lemonade (freshly squeezed preferred)

    Unlimited plain water (flat or fizzy)

    1 cup of flavored water

    1 cup of juice (not from concentrate)

    1 cup of unsweetened iced tea or any other type of tea

    1 cup of low-fat, reduced-fat, or fat-free milk, unsweetened soy milk, or unsweetened almond milk

SNACK 2

- 150 calories or less

MEAL 3

- 1 bowl of soup (no potatoes, no cream). Good choices are chicken noodle, vegetable, lentil, chickpea, split

pea, black bean, tomato bisque, etc. Be careful of sodium content!

- 1 piece of fruit *or* 1 serving of veggies
- Choose one of the following beverages. Choose a different beverage from the one you chose with meal 2.

   One 12-ounce can of diet soda

   1 cup of lemonade (freshly squeezed preferred)

   Unlimited plain water (flat or fizzy)

   1 cup of flavored water

   1 cup of juice (not from concentrate)

   1 cup of unsweetened iced tea or any other type of tea

   1 cup of low-fat, reduced-fat, or fat-free milk, unsweetened soy milk, or unsweetened almond milk

SNACK 3

- 100 calories or less

MEAL 4

- Choose one of the following:

   5-ounce piece of lean beef (no frying)

   5-ounce piece of chicken (no skin, no frying)

   5-ounce piece of fish (no frying)

   5-ounce piece of turkey (no skin, no frying)

   1 cup of spaghetti and meatballs

   (5 ounces is about the size of a deck and a half of
   playing cards.)

- 1 serving of veggies
- Half of a baked sweet potato (no whipped cream or other
  additions; you can add 1 teaspoon of butter) *or* ½ cup of
  rice (brown preferred, but you can have white if you
  choose)

- Choose one of the following beverages. Choose a different beverage from what you chose for meals 2 and 3.

  One 12-ounce can of diet soda

  1 cup of lemonade (freshly squeezed preferred)

  Unlimited plain water (flat or fizzy)

  1 cup of flavored water

  1 cup of juice (not from concentrate)

  1 cup of unsweetened iced tea or any other type of tea

  1 cup of low-fat, reduced-fat, or fat-free milk, unsweetened soy milk, or unsweetened almond milk

EXERCISE

Rest Day. But if you're inspired to do something, by all means go and do it. Every minute of exercise burns more calories and gets you closer to your goal. You might even try playing a sport, which can be a fun way to burn calories without feeling like you're actually working out.

SHRED WEEK 3, DAY 5

MEAL 1

- 1 cup of lemon water. Pour 8 ounces of water, either hot or cold. Squeeze the juice from half a lemon directly into the water. If you prefer, add ½ teaspoon of sugar. Mix well and drink.

- Choose one of the following. Your choice must be 200 calories or less and no sugar added.

  1 fruit smoothie

    1 protein shake

    1 veggie shake

SNACK 1

- 150 calories or less

MEAL 2

- Choose one of the following. Your choice must be less than 300 calories and no sugar added. Try to choose something different from your choice for meal 1.

    1 fruit smoothie

    1 protein shake

    1 veggie shake

- 1 piece of fruit *or* 1 serving of veggies
- Choose one of the following beverages:

    One 12-ounce can of diet soda

    1 cup of lemonade (freshly squeezed preferred)

    Unlimited plain water (flat or fizzy)

    1 cup of flavored water

    1 cup of juice (not from concentrate)

    1 cup of unsweetened iced tea or any other type of tea

    1 cup of low-fat, reduced-fat, or fat-free milk, unsweetened soy milk, or unsweetened almond milk

SNACK 2

- 150 calories or less

MEAL 3

- 1 small green garden salad (Only 3 tablespoons of fat-free dressing, no bacon bits, no croutons. Keep it clean.)

- 1 chicken or turkey sandwich on 100-percent whole-wheat or 100-percent whole-grain bread; lettuce, tomato, 1 slice of cheese, and 1 teaspoon of mustard or mayo if desired. (You can always substitute a medium salad for a meal. Just remember only 3 tablespoons of fat-free dressing, no bacon bits, no croutons. Keep it clean.)
- Choose one of the following beverages. Choose a different beverage from the one you chose in meal 2.

  One 12-ounce can of diet soda

  1 cup of lemonade (freshly squeezed preferred)

  Unlimited plain water (flat or fizzy)

  1 cup of flavored water

  1 cup of juice (not from concentrate)

  1 cup of unsweetened iced tea or any other type of tea

  1 cup of low-fat, reduced-fat, or fat-free milk, unsweetened soy milk, or unsweetened almond milk

SNACK 3

- 150 calories or less

MEAL 4

- Choose one of the following. Your choice must be 200 calories or less and no sugar added. Try to choose something different from what you chose for meal 2.

  1 fruit smoothie

  1 protein shake

  1 veggie shake

  1 bowl of soup (no potatoes, no cream). Good choices are chicken noodle, vegetable, lentil, chickpea, split

> pea, black bean, tomato bisque, etc. Be careful of sodium content!

- 1 serving of fruit *or* 1 serving of veggies
- Choose one of the following beverages. Choose a different beverage from what you chose with meals 2 and 3.

   One 12-ounce can of diet soda

   1 cup of lemonade (freshly squeezed preferred)

   Unlimited plain water (flat or fizzy)

   1 cup of flavored water

   1 cup of juice (not from concentrate)

   1 cup of unsweetened iced tea or any other type of tea

   1 cup of low-fat, reduced-fat, or fat-free milk, unsweetened soy milk, or unsweetened almond milk

SNACK 4

- 100 calories or less

EXERCISE

- Amount of exercise today: Minimum 40 minutes. If you want to do more, all the better! Work as hard as you can!
- Choose from this list of cardiovascular exercises. If you need to break up the time into two workout sessions, that's completely acceptable. What's most important is that you actually perform the exercise for the minimum amount of time indicated. Work hard!

   Jogging outside

   Walking/running on treadmill

   Elliptical machine

   Stationary or mobile bicycle

Swimming laps
Stair climber
225 jump rope revolutions
Treadmill walk/run intervals
Zumba or other type of aerobics
Spinning class
Other high-intensity cardio programs
Rowing machine

SHRED WEEK 3, DAY 6

MEAL 1

- 1 cup of lemon water. Pour 8 ounces of water, either hot or cold. Squeeze the juice of half a lemon directly into the water. If you prefer, add ½ teaspoon of sugar. Mix well and drink.
- 1 piece of fruit
- Choose one of the following:

    1 small bowl of oatmeal (1½ cups cooked)

    2 egg whites *or* 1 egg-white omelet with diced veggies (made with 2 egg whites max)

    1 small bowl of sugar-free cereal with fat-free, skim, or 1-percent fat milk

    1 grilled cheese sandwich on 100-percent whole-grain or 100-percent whole-wheat bread
- 1 cup of fresh juice

SNACK 1

- 100 calories or less

MEAL 2

- Choose one of the following. Your choice must be 200 calories or less.

    1 fruit smoothie

    1 protein shake

    1 veggie shake

    1 bowl of soup (no potatoes, no cream sauces, no meat). Good choices are vegetable, lentil, chickpea, split pea, black bean, tomato bisque, etc. Be careful of sodium content!

- 1 piece of fruit *or* 1 serving of veggies

- Choose one of the following beverages:

    One 12-ounce can of diet soda

    1 cup of lemonade (freshly squeezed preferred)

    Unlimited plain water (flat or fizzy)

    1 cup of flavored water

    1 cup of juice (not from concentrate)

    1 cup of unsweetened iced tea or any other type of tea

    1 cup of low-fat, reduced-fat, or fat-free milk, unsweetened soy milk, or unsweetened almond milk

SNACK 2

- 100 calories or less

MEAL 3

- Choose one of the following. Your choice must be 200 calories or less. Try to choose something different from what you chose in meal 2.

    1 fruit smoothie

    1 protein shake

1 bowl of soup (no potatoes, no cream sauces, no meat). Good choices are vegetable, lentil, chickpea, split pea, black bean, tomato bisque, etc. Be careful of sodium content!

- 1 piece of fruit *or* 1 serving of veggies
- Choose one of the following beverage. Choose a different beverage from what you chose in meal 2.

  One 12-ounce can of diet soda

  1 cup of lemonade (freshly squeezed preferred)

  Unlimited plain water (flat or fizzy)

  1 cup of flavored water

  1 cup of juice (not from concentrate)

  1 cup of unsweetened iced tea or any other type of tea

  1 cup of low-fat, reduced-fat, or fat-free milk, unsweetened soy milk, or unsweetened almond milk

SNACK 3

- 100 calories or less

MEAL 4

- 1 cup of beans (no baked beans)
- Choose one of the following. Your choice must be 200 calories or less. Try to choose something different from what you chose in meal 3.

  1 fruit smoothie

  1 protein shake

  1 veggie shake

- Choose one of the following beverages. Choose a different beverage from the choices with meals 2 and 3.

One 12-ounce can of diet soda

1 cup of lemonade (freshly squeezed preferred)

Unlimited plain water (flat or fizzy)

1 cup of flavored water

1 cup of juice (not from concentrate)

1 cup of unsweetened iced tea or any other type of tea

1 cup of low-fat, reduced-fat, or fat-free milk, unsweetened soy milk, or unsweetened almond milk

SNACK 4

- Choose one of the following:

    20 almonds

    2 rice cakes with 1 teaspoon peanut butter

    Small fruit cup

    8 halves of dried apricots

    2 tablespoons of sunflower seeds

    4 slices of Melba whole-wheat or whole-grain toast

EXERCISE

Rest Day. But if you're inspired to do something, by all means go and do it. Every minute of exercise burns more calories and gets you closer to your goal. You might even try playing a sport, which can be a fun way to burn calories without feeling like you're actually working out.

SHRED WEEK 3, DAY 7

MEAL 1

- 1 cup of lemon water. Pour 8 ounces of water, either hot or cold. Squeeze the juice from half a lemon directly into the water. If you prefer, add ½ teaspoon of sugar. Mix well and drink.
- Choose one of the following. Your choice must be 200 calories or less.

    1 fruit smoothie

    1 protein shake

    1 veggie shake
- 1 piece of fruit

SNACK 1

- 100 calories or less

MEAL 2

- Choose one of the following:

    1 protein shake

    1 veggie shake

    1 bowl of soup (no potatoes, no cream sauces, no meat). Good choices are vegetable, lentil, chickpea, split pea, black bean, tomato bisque, etc. Be careful of sodium content!
- Choose one of the following beverages:

    One 12-ounce can of diet soda

    1 cup of lemonade (freshly squeezed preferred)

    Unlimited plain water (flat or fizzy)

1 cup of flavored water

1 cup of juice (not from concentrate)

1 cup of unsweetened iced tea or any other type of tea

1 cup of low-fat, reduced-fat, or fat-free milk unsweetened soy milk, or unsweetened almond milk

SNACK 2

- 150 calories or less

MEAL 3

- Choose from Group A *or* Group B. *Do not* choose from both.

    Group A—choose one of the following:

    5-ounce piece of chicken (no skin, no frying)

    5-ounce piece of fish (no frying)

    5-ounce piece of turkey (no skin, no frying)

    All of the above come with ½ cup of brown rice and 1 serving of veggies.

    Group B—you can have both items below:

    1 serving of lasagna (with or without meat), 4 inches × 2 inches × 1 inch

    1 serving of veggies

- Choose one of the following beverages. Choose a different beverage from what you chose with meal 2.

    One 12-ounce can of diet soda

    1 cup of lemonade (freshly squeezed preferred)

    Unlimited plain water (flat or fizzy)

    1 cup of flavored water

    1 cup of juice (not from concentrate)

    1 cup of unsweetened iced tea or any other type of tea

1 cup of low-fat, reduced-fat, or fat-free milk, un-sweetened soy milk, or unsweetened almond milk

SNACK 3

- 100 calories or less

MEAL 4

- Choose one of the following. Your choice must be 200 calories or less.

    1 fruit smoothie

    1 protein shake

    1 bowl of soup (no potatoes, no cream). Good choices are chicken noodle, vegetable, lentil, chickpea, split pea, black bean, tomato bisque, etc. Be careful of so-dium content!

- Choose one of the following beverages. Choose a different beverage from what you chose with meals 2 and 3.

    One 12-ounce can of diet soda

    1 cup of lemonade (freshly squeezed preferred)

    Unlimited plain water (flat or fizzy)

    1 cup of flavored water

    1 cup of juice (not from concentrate)

    1 cup of unsweetened iced tea or any other type of tea

    1 cup of low-fat, reduced-fat, or fat-free milk, un-sweetened soy milk, or unsweetened almond milk

EXERCISE

- Amount of exercise today: Minimum 40 minutes. Break up your workout into two sessions. The first session should occur before 12:00 P.M. The second workout should occur after 2:00 P.M. If you want to do more, all the better! Work as hard as you can!

- Choose from this list of cardiovascular exercises. Work hard!

   Jogging outside

   Walking/running on treadmill

   Elliptical machine

   Stationary or mobile bicycle

   Swimming laps

   Stair climber

   225 jump rope revolutions

   Treadmill walk/run intervals

   Zumba or other type of aerobics

   Spinning class

   Other high-intensity cardio programs

   Rowing machine

CHAPTER 6

Week 4: Ascend

Wow! This is spectacular! You have made it to the fourth leg of your journey. You have not only survived, but conquered Transformation, the toughest week in the cycle. After the last seven days, you can do absolutely anything. It's important to visualize what you'll be doing this week. Think about the last three weeks as a descent into a cold, dark pit. Each week you went deeper into the pit. At the end of week 3, you hit bottom. This means it's time to ascend and reach for the light.

Any climber will tell you that a successful ascent requires two things: physical toughness and mental toughness. You have developed both of these attributes over the last few weeks and may not have even known that you were doing so. You will encounter some easy moments along the ascent and some that are quite precarious and exhausting. Ascend week is about combining all that you have learned the last three weeks and employing your knowledge in a way that will get you back to the light. In only seven days you will climb your way out of that dark, lonely pit and make it back on solid ground where you can breathe clean air and enjoy all that's around you. You are now a SHRED veteran, so nothing is too difficult for you to complete. Believe! Work hard! Have fun!

SHRED WEEK 4 GUIDELINES

▶ Weigh yourself in the morning before starting the program and record it. Don't weigh yourself throughout the week. Your next weigh-in will be the same day the following week in the morning. Weigh yourself in the same manner as you did in the beginning. If you weighed in without wearing clothes initially, then do that again. If you weighed in wearing certain clothes, wear the same clothes for the second weigh-in. Use the same scale both times. *Don't* use a different scale as scales can differ by several pounds.

▶ You must eat something every 3 to 4 hours even if you're not hungry, but *don't* stuff yourself. Eat until you're no longer hungry, but *don't eat until you're full.* If you need less than what's recommended, then great, go ahead and eat less, which is even better. Switching meals is permitted, but try to switch as infrequently as possible. For example, if you know that what's listed for meal 3 is easier to get than what's listed for meal 2, then go ahead and switch those meals. Looking at the day's meals in advance is important as it allows you to best prepare for what's ahead.

▶ Five of the seven days you must do some type of cardiovascular exercise, commonly called cardio. Pay attention to the guidelines written for that day. If you need to exercise on different days than listed, then go ahead and do that as long as you get five days of cardio-related physical activity in a seven-day period.

▶ If you don't eat meat, make the substitutions appropriately with fish or vegetables.

▶ This week, all shakes and smoothies are still 200 calories or less. Avoid added sugars if possible in those items that you buy in the store.

▶ When cooking or buying your soups, make sure they are 200 calories or less and low in sodium (salt); this means the sodium or Na+ line on the label should say no more than 480 milligrams per serving. Try eating things made with sea salt as it still gives you the flavor but has less sodium content.

▶ Soups can be consumed with 2 saltine crackers if desired.

▶ The liquid meals must be eaten with either 1 piece of fruit or 1 serving of vegetables.

▶ You must consume 1 cup of water before eating a meal; you must consume 1 cup of water during your meal. You can add lemon or lime to your water, and you can drink fizzy water if you desire.

▶ You are allowed to drink coffee, but only 1 small cup per day. Stay away from all of those fancy coffee preparations that have a lot of calories. Your coffee should contain no more than 50 calories.

▶ Do not eat the last meal within 90 minutes of going to sleep.

▶ You can eat a 100-calorie snack before going to bed if desired.

▶ Be smart in your snack choices. Avoid chips and doughnuts and candy; you can have them some of the time, but don't eat them often. If you must have something like these items, make it only one of your snacks for the day and use healthier options for the other snacks.

▶ You don't have to eat all of the food on the day's menu if you don't want to, but no skipping meals, no doubling up on meals, and no exceeding the meal guidelines in size and volume.

▶ Condiments such as ketchup, mayo, and mustard are allowed, but no more than a teaspoon at each meal. The same goes for soy sauce.

▶ Spices are unlimited.

▶ While fresh fruit is always preferred, canned and frozen fruit are allowed. Just make sure they are water-based and there are no added sugars.

▶ Canned and frozen vegetables are allowed. Please be aware of the sodium content.

▶ As far as beverages are concerned, you are allowed as much water as you like per day. Here are some other beverage guidelines:

No regular soda

One 12-ounce can of diet soda allowed each day

Flavored waters allowed, but keep them under 60 calories

1 bottle of sports drink allowed per day, but keep under 60 calories

For alcohol, 1 mixed drink allowed twice a week, *or* 3 light beers allowed per week, *or* 3 regular glasses of wine (red or white) allowed per week

Timing is critical to the success of this plan. It might be difficult at first, but plan in advance and do the best you can. Skipping meals is not advised. Even if you eat just a small portion, try to eat something on schedule.

A sample day's schedule during Ascend might look something like the grid below, but for each and every day, the order of the meals and snacks is both intended and critical. And on some days, there's a bonus fourth snack, so follow each day's directions carefully.

8:30 A.M.	10:00 A.M.	11:30 A.M.	1:00 P.M.	3:30 P.M.	7:00 P.M.	8:30 P.M.
Meal 1	Snack 1	Meal 2	Snack 2	Meal 3	Meal 4	Snack 3

SHRED WEEK 4, DAY 1

MEAL 1

- 1 cup of lemon water. Pour 8 ounces of water, either hot or cold. Squeeze the juice from half of lemon directly into the water. If you prefer, add ½ teaspoon of sugar. Mix well and drink.
- 1 piece of fruit. This can be 1 banana, 1 apple, 1 pear, etc. It can also be ½ cup of raspberries, blueberries, blackberries, or strawberries.
- Choose only one of the following.
    1 small bowl of oatmeal (1–1½ cups cooked)
    2 egg whites *or* 1 egg-white omelet with diced veggies (made with 2 egg whites max)
    1 small bowl of sugar-free cereal with fat-free, skim, or 1-percent fat milk
- ½ cup of juice *not* from concentrate (grapefruit, apple, orange, carrot, pear, tomato, etc.)

SNACK 1

- 100 calories or less

MEAL 2

- 1 chicken or turkey sandwich on 100-percent whole-wheat or 100-percent whole-grain bread; lettuce, tomato, 1 slice of cheese, and 1 teaspoon of mustard or mayo if desired
- 1 small green garden salad (Only 3 tablespoons of fat-free dressing, no bacon bits, no croutons. Keep it clean.)
- Choose one of the following beverages:

    One 12-ounce can of diet soda

    1 cup of lemonade (freshly squeezed preferred)

    Unlimited plain water (flat or fizzy)

    1 cup of flavored water

    1 cup of juice (not from concentrate)

    1 cup of unsweetened iced tea

    1 cup of low-fat, reduced-fat, or fat-free milk, unsweetened soy milk, or unsweetened almond milk

SNACK 2

- 100 calories or less

MEAL 3

- Choose one of the following. Your choice must not exceed 200 calories.

    1 milk shake

    1 fruit smoothie

    1 protein shake

    1 veggie shake (You can use any veggies you want.)

1 bowl of soup (no potatoes, no cream). Good choices are chicken noodle, vegetable, lentil, chickpea, split pea, black bean, tomato bisque, etc. Be careful of sodium content!

- Choose one of the following beverages. Choose a different beverage from your choice in meal 2.

    One 12-ounce can of diet soda

    1 cup of lemonade (freshly squeezed preferred)

    Unlimited plain water (flat or fizzy)

    1 cup of flavored water

    1 cup of juice (not from concentrate)

    1 cup of unsweetened iced tea

MEAL 4

- Choose one item from Group A *and* one item from Group B

    Group A

    1 small bowl of pasta with marinara sauce (*no cream sauces*)

    2 small-to-medium slices of pizza (triangular cut: 4 inches width across crust, 6 inches in length)

    1 cheeseburger or hamburger (3½ inches in diameter, ½-inch thick)

    1 bowl of soup (no potatoes, no cream). Good choices are chicken noodle, vegetable, lentil, chickpea, split pea, black bean, tomato bisque, etc. Be careful of sodium content!

    5-ounce piece of turkey (no skin, no frying)

    5-ounce piece of chicken (no skin, no frying)

    5-ounce piece of fish (no frying)

Group B

French fries (about 12 skinny fries or 6 steak fries)

1 serving of veggies

Small green garden salad

- Choose one of the following beverages:

  One 12-ounce can of diet soda

  1 cup of lemonade (freshly squeezed preferred)

  Unlimited plain water (flat or fizzy)

  1 cup of flavored water

  1 cup of juice (not from concentrate)

  1 cup of unsweetened iced tea

SNACK 3

- 100 calories or less

EXERCISE

- Amount of exercise today: Minimum 30 minutes. If you want to do more, all the better! Work as hard as you can!
- Choose a combination of the items below to fulfill your exercise requirement:

  15 minutes jogging outside

  15 minutes walking/running on treadmill

  15 minutes on elliptical machine

  15 minutes on stationary or mobile bicycle

  15 minutes swimming laps

  15 minutes on stair climber

  225 jump rope revolutions

  20 minutes treadmill intervals

  15 minutes of Zumba

15 minutes of spinning

15 minutes of any other high-intensity cardio

15 minutes of rowing machine

SHRED WEEK 4, DAY 2

MEAL 1

- 1 cup of lemon water. Pour 8 ounces of water, either hot or cold. Squeeze the juice of half a lemon directly into the water. If you like, add ½ teaspoon of sugar. Mix well and drink.

- Choose one of the following. Your choice must not exceed 200 calories.

    1 milk shake (must be made with low-fat or skim milk)

    1 fruit smoothie

    1 protein shake

    1 veggie smoothie (You can use any veggies you want.)

- 1 piece of fruit

SNACK 1

- 100 calories or less

MEAL 2

- Choose one of the following:

    3 servings of vegetables (Remember, a serving is about the size of the average person's fist.)

    1 large green garden salad (no croutons, no bacon bits, 4 tablespoons of fat-free or low-fat dressing)

      1 fruit smoothie (200 calories or less)

      1 protein shake (200 calories or less)

- Choose one of the following beverages:

      One 12-ounce can of diet soda

      1 cup of lemonade (freshly squeezed preferred)

      Unlimited plain water (flat or fizzy)

      1 cup of flavored water

      1 cup of juice (not from concentrate)

      1 cup of unsweetened iced tea

SNACK 2

- 150 calories or less

MEAL 3

- Choose one of the following. Your choice should be different from your selection for meal 2.

      3 servings of vegetables (Remember, a serving is about the size of the average person's fist.)

      1 large green garden salad (no croutons, no bacon bits, 4 tablespoons of fat-free or low-fat dressing)

      1 fruit smoothie (200 calories or less)

      1 protein shake (200 calories or less)

- Choose one of the following beverages. Your choice must be different from the beverage chosen for meal 2.

      One 12-ounce can of diet soda

      1 cup of lemonade (freshly squeezed preferred)

      Unlimited plain water (flat or fizzy)

      1 cup of flavored water

      1 cup of juice (not from concentrate)

      1 cup of unsweetened iced tea

SNACK 3

- 100 calories or less

MEAL 4

- Choose one of the following. Your choice should be different from your selection for meal 3.

  3 servings of vegetables (Remember, a serving is about the size of the average person's fist.)

  1 large green garden salad (no croutons, no bacon bits, 4 tablespoons of fat-free or low-fat dressing)

  1 veggie burger (3½ inches in diameter, ½-inch thick)

  1 protein shake (200 calories or less)

  1 bowl of soup (200 calories or less; no potatoes, no cream). Good choices are chicken noodle, vegetable, lentil, chickpea, split pea, black bean, tomato bisque, etc. Be careful of sodium content!

- If you choose the protein shake or soup, you should also consume 1 serving of veggies

- Choose one of the following beverages. Your choice must be different from the beverage chosen for meals 2 and 3.

  One 12-ounce can of diet soda

  1 cup of lemonade (freshly squeezed preferred)

  Unlimited plain water (flat or fizzy)

  1 cup of flavored water

  1 cup of juice (not from concentrate)

  1 cup of unsweetened iced tea

EXERCISE

- Amount of exercise today: Minimum 45 minutes. If you want to do more, all the better! Work as hard as you can!

- Choose a combination of the items below to fulfill your exercise requirement:

   15 minutes jogging outside

   15 minutes walking/running on treadmill

   15 minutes on elliptical machine

   15 minutes on stationary or mobile bicycle

   15 minutes swimming laps

   15 minutes on stair climber

   225 jump rope revolutions

   20 minutes treadmill intervals

   15 minutes of Zumba

   15 minutes spinning

   15 minutes of any other high-intensity cardio

   15 minutes of rowing machine

SHRED WEEK 4, DAY 3

MEAL 1

- 1 cup of lemon water. Pour 8 ounces of water, either hot or cold. Squeeze the juice of half a lemon directly into the water. If you like, add ½ teaspoon of sugar. Mix well and drink.
- 1 piece of fruit. This can be 1 banana, 1 apple, 1 pear, etc. It can also be ½ cup of raspberries, blueberries, blackberries, or strawberries.
- Choose one of the following. Your portion should be 1 cup cooked.

   1 small bowl of oatmeal

1 small bowl of Cream of Wheat

1 small bowl of grits

- 1 cup of juice *not* from concentrate (grapefruit, apple, orange, carrot, pear, tomato, etc.)

SNACK 1

- 100 calories or less

MEAL 2

- Choose one of the following. Your choice must be 200 calories or less.

  1 fruit smoothie

  1 protein shake

  1 bowl of soup (no potatoes, no cream). Good choices are chicken noodle, vegetable, lentil, chickpea, split pea, black bean, tomato bisque, etc. Be careful of sodium content!

- 1 piece of fruit *or* 1 serving of veggies
- Choose one of the following beverages:

  One 12-ounce can of diet soda

  1 cup of lemonade (freshly squeezed preferred)

  Unlimited plain water (flat or fizzy)

  1 cup of flavored water

  1 cup of juice (not from concentrate)

  1 cup of unsweetened iced tea

SNACK 2

- 150 calories or less

MEAL 3

- Choose one of the following. Your choice must not exceed 200 calories. Try to choose something different

from what you had in meal 2 if you can. You don't
have to, but try.

　1 milk shake

　1 fruit smoothie

　1 protein shake

　1 veggie shake (You can use any veggies you want.)

　1 bowl of soup (no potatoes, no cream). Good choices
　are chicken noodle, vegetable, lentil, chickpea, split
　pea, black bean, tomato bisque, etc. Be careful of so-
　dium content!

- Choose one of the following. Choose something different from what was chosen with meal 2.

　One 12-ounce can of diet soda

　1 cup of lemonade (freshly squeezed preferred)

　Unlimited plain water (flat or fizzy)

　1 cup of flavored water

　1 cup of juice (not from concentrate)

　1 cup of unsweetened iced tea

SNACK 3

- 100 calories or less

MEAL 4

- Choose from Group A *or* Group B. *Do not* choose from
  both.

　Group A—choose one of the following:

　　5-ounce piece of chicken (no skin, no frying)

　　5-ounce piece of fish (no frying)

　　5-ounce piece of turkey (no skin, no frying)

　All of the above come with ½ cup of brown rice and
　1 serving of veggies.

Group B—you can have both items below:

1 serving of lasagna (with or without meat), 4 inches × 2 1 inch

1 serving of veggies

- Choose one of the following beverages. Choose something different from what was chosen with meal 3.

One 12-ounce can of diet soda

1 cup of lemonade (freshly squeezed preferred)

Unlimited plain water (flat or fizzy)

1 cup of flavored water

1 cup of juice (not from concentrate)

1 cup of unsweetened iced tea

EXERCISE

Rest Day. But if you're inspired to do something, by all means go and do it. Every minute of exercise burns more calories and gets you closer to your goal. You might even try playing a sport, which can be a fun way to burn calories without feeling like you're actually working out.

SHRED WEEK 4, DAY 4

MEAL 1

- 1 cup of lemon water. Pour 8 ounces of water, either hot or cold. Squeeze the juice from half a lemon directly into the water. If you like, add ½ teaspoon of sugar. Mix well and drink.
- 1 cup of raspberries, sliced strawberries, blueberries, or blackberries

- Choose one of the following. Your choice must be 200 calories or less and no sugar added.

    1 fruit smoothie

    1 protein shake
- ½ cup of juice *not* from concentrate (grapefruit, apple, orange, carrot, pear, tomato, etc.)

SNACK 1

- 100 calories or less

MEAL 2

- Choose one of the following:

    3 servings of vegetables (Remember, a serving is about the size of the average person's fist.)

    1 large green garden salad (no croutons, no bacon bits, 4 tablespoons of fat-free or low-fat dressing)

    1 veggie burger (3½ inches in diameter, ½-inch thick)

    1 protein shake (200 calories or less)

    1 bowl of soup (200 calories or less; no potatoes, no cream). Good choices are chicken noodle, vegetable, lentil, chickpea, split pea, black bean, tomato bisque, etc. Be careful of sodium content!
- If you choose the protein shake or soup, you should also consume 1 serving of veggies.
- Choose one of the following beverages:

    One 12-ounce can of diet soda

    1 cup of lemonade (freshly squeezed preferred)

    Unlimited plain water (flat or fizzy)

    1 cup of flavored water

    1 cup of juice (not from concentrate)

    1 cup of unsweetened iced tea

1 cup of low-fat, reduced-fat, or fat-free milk, unsweetened soy milk, or unsweetened almond milk

SNACK 2

- 150 calories or less

MEAL 3

- Choose one of the following:

  5-ounce piece of lean beef (no frying)

  5-ounce piece of chicken (no skin, no frying)

  5-ounce piece of fish (no frying)

  5-ounce piece of turkey (no skin, no frying)

  1 cup of spaghetti and meatballs

  (5 ounces is about the size of a deck and a half of playing cards.)
- 1 serving of veggies
- Half of a baked sweet potato (no whipped cream or other additions; you can add 1 teaspoon of butter) *or* ½ cup of rice (brown preferred, but you can have white if you choose)
- Choose one of the following beverages. Choose a different beverage from what you chose for meal 2.

  One 12-ounce can of diet soda

  1 cup of lemonade (freshly squeezed preferred)

  Unlimited plain water (flat or fizzy)

  1 cup of flavored water

  1 cup of juice (not from concentrate)

  1 cup of unsweetened iced tea

  1 cup of low-fat, reduced-fat, or fat-free milk, unsweetened soy milk, or unsweetened almond milk

SNACK 3

- 100 calories or less

MEAL 4

- Choose one of the following. Your choice must be 200 calories or less and no sugar added.

    1 fruit smoothie

    1 protein shake

    1 veggie smoothie

- Choose one of the following beverages. Choose a different beverage from what you chose for meal 3.

    One 12-ounce can of diet soda

    1 cup of lemonade (freshly squeezed preferred)

    Unlimited plain water (flat or fizzy)

    1 cup of flavored water

    1 cup of juice (not from concentrate)

    1 cup of unsweetened iced tea

    1 cup of low-fat, reduced-fat, or fat-free milk, unsweetened soy milk, or unsweetened almond milk

EXERCISE

- Amount of exercise today: Minimum 30 minutes. If you want to do more, all the better! Work as hard as you can!

- Choose a combination of the items below to fulfill your exercise requirement:

    15 minutes jogging outside

    15 minutes walking/running on treadmill

    15 minutes on elliptical machine

    15 minutes on stationary or mobile bicycle

15 minutes swimming laps

15 minutes on stair climber

225 jump rope revolutions

20 minutes treadmill intervals

15 minutes of Zumba

15 minutes of spinning

15 minutes of any other high-intensity cardio

15 minutes of rowing machine

SHRED WEEK 4, DAY 5

MEAL 1

- 1 cup of lemon water. Pour 8 ounces of water, either hot or cold. Squeeze the juice from half a lemon directly into the water. If you like, add ½ teaspoon of sugar. Mix well and drink.
- Choose one of the following. Your choice must be 200 calories or less and no sugar added.

    1 fruit smoothie

    1 protein shake

    1 veggie shake

SNACK 1

- 150 calories or less

MEAL 2

- Choose one of the following:

    2 chicken fingers

    Chicken stir-fry (1 cup)

　　　5-ounce piece of fish (not fried)

　　　6 jumbo shrimp (2 tablespoons cocktail sauce)

　　　1 cup of pasta (no cream sauce)

　　　3 servings of veggies

- 1 serving of veggies if you did not choose veggies above.

- Choose one of the following beverages:

　　　One 12-ounce can of diet soda

　　　1 cup of lemonade (freshly squeezed preferred)

　　　Unlimited plain water (flat or fizzy)

　　　1 cup of flavored water

　　　1 cup of juice (not from concentrate)

　　　1 cup of unsweetened iced tea or 2 cups of any other kind of tea

　　　1 cup of low-fat, reduced-fat, or fat-free milk, unsweetened soy milk, or unsweetened almond milk

SNACK 2

- 150 calories or less

MEAL 3

- Choose one of the following. Your choice must be 200 calories or less and no sugar added.

　　　1 fruit smoothie

　　　1 protein shake

　　　1 veggie shake

- 1 serving of veggies

- Choose one of the following beverages. Choose a different beverage from what you chose with meal 2.

　　　One 12-ounce can of diet soda

　　　1 cup of lemonade (freshly squeezed preferred)

Unlimited plain water (flat or fizzy)

1 cup of flavored water

1 cup of juice (not from concentrate)

1 cup of unsweetened iced tea or 2 cups of any other type of tea

1 cup of low-fat, reduced-fat, or fat-free milk, unsweetened soy milk, or unsweetened almond milk

SNACK 3

- 150 calories or less

MEAL 4

- Choose one of the following:

    5-ounce piece of lean beef (no frying)

    5-ounce piece of chicken (no skin, no frying)

    5-ounce piece of fish (no frying)

    5-ounce piece of turkey (no skin, no frying)

    One cup of spaghetti and meatballs

    (5 ounces is about the size of a deck and a half of playing cards.)

- 1 serving of veggies

- Half of a baked sweet potato (no whipped cream or other additions; you can add 1 teaspoon of butter) *or* ½ cup of rice (brown preferred, but you can have white if you wish)

- Choose one of the following. Choose a different beverage from what you chose for meal 3.

    One 12-ounce can of diet soda

    1 cup of lemonade (freshly squeezed preferred)

    Unlimited plain water (flat or fizzy)

    1 cup of flavored water

1 cup of juice (not from concentrate)

1 cup of unsweetened iced tea or 2 cups of any other type of tea

1 cup of low-fat, reduced-fat, or fat-free milk, unsweetened soy milk, or unsweetened almond milk

SNACK 4

- 100 calories or less

EXERCISE

- Amount of exercise today: Minimum 45 minutes. If you want to do more, all the better! Work as hard as you can!
- Choose a combination of the items below to fulfill your exercise requirement:

  15 minutes jogging outside

  15 minutes walking/running on treadmill

  15 minutes on elliptical machine

  15 minutes on stationary or mobile bicycle

  15 minutes swimming laps

  15 minutes on stair climber

  225 jump rope revolutions

  20 minutes treadmill intervals

  15 minutes of Zumba

  15 minutes of spinning

  15 minutes of any other high-intensity cardio

  15 minutes of rowing machine

SHRED WEEK 4, DAY 6

MEAL 1

- 1 cup of lemon water. Pour 8 ounces of water, either hot or cold. Squeeze the juice from half a lemon directly into the water. If you like, add ½ teaspoon of sugar. Mix well and drink.
- 1 piece of fruit
- Choose one of the following:

    1 small bowl of oatmeal (1 ½ cups cooked)

    2 egg whites *or* 1 egg-white omelet with diced veggies (made with 2 egg whites max)

    1 small bowl of sugar-free cereal with fat-free, skim, or 1-percent fat milk

    1 grilled cheese sandwich on 100-percent whole-grain or 100-percent whole-wheat bread

- 1 cup of juice *not* from concentrate (grapefruit, apple, orange, carrot, pear, tomato, etc.)

SNACK 1

- 100 calories or less

MEAL 2

- Choose one of the following. Your choice must be 200 calories or less.

    1 fruit smoothie

    1 protein shake

    1 veggie shake

    1 bowl of soup (no potatoes, no cream, no meat).

Good choices are vegetable, lentil, chickpea, split pea, black bean, tomato bisque, etc. Be careful of sodium content!

- 1 piece of fruit *or* 1 serving of veggies
- Choose one of the following beverages:

    One 12-ounce can of diet soda

    1 cup of lemonade (freshly squeezed preferred)

    Unlimited plain water (flat or fizzy)

    1 cup of flavored water

    1 cup of juice (not from concentrate)

    1 cup of unsweetened iced tea or 2 cups of any other type of tea

    1 cup of low-fat, reduced-fat, or fat-free milk, unsweetened soy milk, or unsweetened almond milk

SNACK 2

- 100 calories or less

MEAL 3

- Choose one of the following. Your choice must be 200 calories or less. Try to choose something different from what you chose for meal 2.

    1 fruit smoothie

    1 protein shake

    1 bowl of soup (no potatoes, no cream, no meat). Good choices are vegetable, lentil, chickpea, split pea, black bean, tomato bisque, etc. Be careful of sodium content!

- 1 piece of fruit *or* 1 serving of veggies
- Choose one of the following beverages. Choose a different one from what you chose for meal 2.

One 12-ounce can of diet soda

1 cup of lemonade (freshly squeezed preferred)

Unlimited plain water (flat or fizzy)

1 cup of flavored water

1 cup of juice (not from concentrate)

1 cup of unsweetened iced tea or 2 cups of any other type of tea

1 cup of low-fat, reduced-fat, or fat-free milk, unsweetened soy milk, or unsweetened almond milk

SNACK 3

- 100 calories or less

MEAL 4

- 1 cup of beans (no baked beans)
- Choose one of the following. Your choice must be 200 calories or less. Try to choose something different from what you chose for meal 3.

    1 fruit smoothie

    1 protein shake

    1 veggie shake

- Choose one of the following beverages. Choose a different beverage from what you chose for meals 2 and 3.

    One 12-ounce can of diet soda

    1 cup of lemonade (freshly squeezed preferred)

    Unlimited plain water (flat or fizzy)

    1 cup of flavored water

    1 cup of juice (not from concentrate)

    1 cup of unsweetened iced tea or 2 cups of any other type of tea

1 cup of low-fat, reduced-fat, or fat-free milk, unsweetened soy milk, or unsweetened almond milk

SNACK 4

- Choose one of the following:

  20 almonds

  2 rice cakes with 2 teaspoons peanut butter

  Small fruit cup

  8 halves of dried apricots

  2 tablespoons of sunflower seeds

  4 slices of Melba whole-wheat or whole-grain toast

  1 large cucumber sliced with 2 tablespoons of fat-free dressing

  1 scoop of ice cream (no more than ½ cup)

EXERCISE

- Rest Day. But if you're inspired to do something, by all means go and do it. Every minute of exercise burns more calories and gets you closer to your goal. You might even try playing a sport, which can be a fun way to burn calories without feeling like you're actually working out.

SHRED WEEK 4, DAY 7

MEAL 1

- 1 cup of lemon water. Pour 8 ounces of water, either hot or cold. Squeeze the juice from half a lemon directly into the water. If you like, add ½ teaspoon of sugar. Mix well and drink.

- Choose one of the following. Your choice must be 200 calories or less.
    1 fruit smoothie
    1 protein shake
    1 veggie shake
- 1 piece of fruit

SNACK 1

- 100 calories or less

MEAL 2

- Choose one of the following. Your choice must be 200 calories or less.
    1 protein shake
    1 veggie shake
    1 bowl of soup (no potatoes, no cream, no meat). Good choices are vegetable, lentil, chickpea, split pea, black bean, tomato bisque, etc. Be careful of sodium content!
- Choose one of the following beverages:
    One 12-ounce can of diet soda
    1 cup of lemonade (freshly squeezed preferred)
    Unlimited plain water (flat or fizzy)
    1 cup of flavored water
    1 cup of juice (not from concentrate)
    1 cup of unsweetened iced tea or 2 cups of any other type of tea
    1 cup of low-fat, reduced-fat, or fat-free milk, unsweetened soy milk, or unsweetened almond milk

SNACK 2

- 150 calories or less

MEAL 3

- Choose from Group A or Group B. *Do not* choose from both.

    Group A—choose one of the following:

    5-ounce piece of chicken (no skin, no frying)

    5-ounce piece of fish (no frying)

    5-ounce piece of turkey (no skin, no frying)

    All of the above come with ½ cup of brown rice and 1 serving of veggies.

    Group B—you can have both items below:

    1 serving of lasagna (with or without meat), 4 inches × 2 inches × 1 inch

    1 serving of veggies

- Choose one of the following beverages. Choose a different beverage from what you chose for meal 2.

    One 12-ounce can of diet soda

    1 cup of lemonade (freshly squeezed preferred)

    Unlimited plain water (flat or fizzy)

    1 cup of flavored water

    1 cup of juice (not from concentrate)

    1 cup of unsweetened iced tea or 2 cups of any other type of tea

    1 cup of low-fat, reduced-fat, or fat-free milk, unsweetened soy milk, or unsweetened almond milk

SNACK 3

- 100 calories or less

MEAL 4

- Choose one of the following. Your choice must be 200 calories or less.

  1 fruit smoothie

  1 protein shake

  1 bowl of soup (no potatoes, no cream). Good choices are chicken noodle, vegetable, lentil, chickpea, split pea, black bean, tomato bisque, etc. Be careful of sodium content!

- Choose one of the following beverages. Choose a different beverage from what you chose for meals 2 and 3.

  One 12-ounce can of diet soda

  1 cup of lemonade (freshly squeezed preferred)

  Unlimited plain water (flat or fizzy)

  1 cup of flavored water

  1 cup of juice (not from concentrate)

  1 cup of unsweetened iced tea or 2 cups of any other type of tea

  1 cup of low-fat, reduced-fat, or fat-free milk, unsweetened soy milk, or unsweetened almond milk

EXERCISE

- Amount of exercise today: Minimum 45 minutes. Break this up into two sessions. Your first session must occur before 12:00 P.M. Your second session can occur any time after 2:00 P.M. If you want to do more, all the better! Work as hard as you can!

- Choose a combination of the items below to fulfill your exercise requirement:

  15 minutes jogging outside

  15 minutes walking/running on treadmill

15 minutes on elliptical machine

15 minutes on stationary or mobile bicycle

15 minutes swimming laps

15 minutes on stair climber

225 jump rope revolutions

20 minutes treadmill intervals

15 minutes of Zumba

15 minutes of spinning

15 minutes of any other high-intensity cardio

15 minutes of rowing machine

CHAPTER 7

Week 5: Cleanse

Welcome back! Congratulations on your ascent. You have not only traveled to the depths in Transformation, but you were able to re-emerge stronger, mentally tougher, and lighter in Ascend. Now that you are no longer in the pit, it's time to Cleanse your body so that you are now one with the fresh air you're breathing.

Almost everyone has heard of the concept of detoxing or cleansing. Done correctly, detoxing can not only be a rewarding experience, but excellent for your health. Some cleanses last as long as thirty days, some as short as a few days. The SHRED cleanse is seven days, enough to give you a fresh start, but not so long that it becomes exhausting and too difficult to follow.

The previous four weeks had various elements of cleansing as part of the regimen. However, this week is a more concentrated effort that will not only cleanse your system, but help you lose weight. The liver is the biggest cleansing organ in our body. It is primarily responsible for removing toxins from your bloodstream and breaking them down so that they can be eliminated. The SHRED cleanse has you eating particular foods and drinking certain beverages that naturally activate enzymes in the liver to enhance the detoxification process. Some programs that call themselves detoxes or cleanses are actually fasts—programs that dramatically reduce what you eat and the calories you consume. These programs can be dangerous if they do not supply you with the proper amount of vitamins, minerals, and nutrients you need to be well nourished and operate at maximal capacity. The SHRED cleanse is an "eating detox," which means you don't go hungry, you're not starved for vitamins or nutrients, and you eat foods that naturally cleanse your body.

You will feel your body make adjustments as it cleanses, so don't be surprised. Your gastrointestinal tract will move better, your energy levels will increase, and your skin will even appear healthier (some have said that it takes on a certain glow). It's important that you really stick as closely to the plan this week as possible. I chose the foods and beverages for specific reasons, so substitute infrequently. Read the guidelines for this chapter closely as there are significant modifications that you must implement. Open your palate and try different foods, and remember: it's only seven days. You've already been to the depths and survived. You can do *anything*, especially a simple *Cleanse*. Believe! Work hard! Have fun!

SHRED WEEK 5 GUIDELINES

▶ Weigh yourself in the morning before starting the program and record it. Don't weigh yourself throughout the week. Your next weigh-in will be the same day the following week in the morning. Weigh yourself in the same manner as you did in the beginning. If you weighed in without wearing clothes initially, then do that again. If you weighed in wearing certain clothes, wear the same clothes for the second weigh-in. Use the same scale both times. *Don't* use a different scale as scales can differ by several pounds.

▶ You must eat something every 3 to 4 hours even if you're not hungry, but *don't* stuff yourself. Eat until you're no longer hungry, but *don't eat until you're full.* If you need less than what's recommended, then great, go ahead and eat less, which is even better. Switching meals is permitted, but try to switch as infrequently as possible. For example, if you know that what's listed for meal 3 is easier to get than what's listed for meal 2, then go ahead and switch them. Looking at the day's meals in advance is important as it allows you to best prepare for what's ahead.

NEW THIS WEEK

1. You must continue to drink lemon water every morning for breakfast, but you will be adding ground flaxseed or flaxseed oil to the water.
2. One cup of hibiscus tea must be consumed every day. If you purchase hibiscus tea that's already been made, make sure that it is 100-percent natural.
3. One cup of 100-percent pure cranberry juice must be consumed every day. You can

dilute the cranberry juice with some water to help cut the bitterness.

4. No alcohol is allowed this week. You will be able to drink again if you like after these seven days, but for these seven days, we need to give your liver a rest from alcohol.

5. In previous weeks you have had the flexibility to choose snacks that you prefer that fit the calorie guidelines. This week you *must* choose snacks from the suggested list. These are specific snacks that assist in the cleanse and increase energy. Be open-minded and experiment with some of the things on the list that you might not have ever tried in the past.

6. This week, shakes and smoothies are different. Some will be only 200 calories while others can be more. Pay attention to the specific guidelines for that meal. Avoid added sugars if possible in those items that you buy in the store.

7. When cooking or buying your soups, note that some will be only 200 calories while others can be more. Pay attention to the specific guidelines for that meal. Make sure they are low in sodium (salt); this means the sodium or Na+ line on the label should say no more than 480 milligrams per serving. Try eating things made with sea salt as it still gives you the flavor, but has less sodium content.

▶ Five of the seven days you must do some type of cardiovascular exercise, commonly called cardio. Pay attention to the guidelines written for that day. If you need to exercise on different days than listed, then go ahead and do that as long as you get five days of cardio-related physical activity in a seven-day period.

▶ If you don't eat meat, make the substitutions appropriately with fish or vegetables.

▶ Soups can be consumed with 2 saltine crackers if desired.

▶ The liquid meals must be eaten with either 1 piece of fruit *or* 1 serving of vegetables.

▶ You must consume 1 cup of water before eating a meal; you must consume 1 cup of water during your meal. You can add lemon or lime to your water and you can drink fizzy water if you desire.

▶ You are allowed to drink coffee, but only 1 small cup per day. Stay away from all of those fancy coffee preparations that have lots of calories. Your coffee should contain no more than 50 calories

▶ Do not eat the last meal within 90 minutes of going to sleep.

▶ You can eat a 100-calorie snack before going to bed if desired.

▶ Be smart in your snack choices. Avoid chips and doughnuts and candy; you can have them some of the time, but don't eat them often. If you must have something like these items, make it only one of your snacks for the day and use healthier options for the other snacks.

▶ You don't have to eat all of the food on the day's menu if you don't want to, but no skipping meals, no doubling up on meals, and no exceeding the meal guidelines in size and volume.

▶ Condiments such as ketchup, mayo, and mustard are allowed, but no more than a teaspoon at each meal. The same goes for soy sauce.

▶ Spices are unlimited.

▶ While fresh fruit is always preferred, canned and frozen fruit are allowed. Just make sure they are water-based and there are no added sugars.

▶ Canned and frozen vegetables are allowed. Please be aware of the sodium content.

▶ As far as beverages are concerned, you are allowed as much water as you like per day. Here are some other beverage guidelines:

No regular soda
One 12-ounce can of diet soda allowed each day
Flavored waters allowed, but keep them under 60 calories
1 bottle of sports drink allowed per day, but keep it under 60 calories
No alcohol

Timing is critical to the success of this plan. It might be difficult at first, but plan in advance and do the best you can. Skipping meals is not advised. Even if you eat just a small portion, try to eat something on schedule. A sample day's schedule during Cleanse might look something like the grid below, but for each and every day, the order of the meals and snacks is both intended and critical. And on some days, there's a bonus fourth snack, so follow each day's directions carefully.

8:30 A.M.	10:00 A.M.	11:30 A.M.	1:00 P.M.	3:30 P.M.	7:00 P.M.	8:30 P.M.
Meal 1	Snack 1	Meal 2	Snack 2	Meal 3	Meal 4	Snack 3

SHRED WEEK 5, DAY 1

MEAL 1

- 1 cup of lemon water. Pour 8 ounces of water, either hot or cold. Squeeze the juice from half a lemon directly into the water. Add 2 tablespoons of ground flaxseeds or flaxseed oil. Mix well and drink.
- 1 piece of fruit. This can be 1 banana, 1 apple, 1 pear, etc. It can also be ½ cup of raspberries, blueberries, blackberries, or strawberries.
- Choose one of the following:

   1 small bowl of oatmeal (1 ½ cups cooked)

   2 egg whites *or* 1 egg-white omelet with diced veggies (made with 2 egg whites max)

   1 small bowl of sugar-free cereal with fat-free, skim, or 1-percent fat milk
- ½ cup of fresh juice *not* from concentrate (grapefruit, apple, orange juice, tomato, carrot, etc.)

SNACK 1

- 100 calories or less

MEAL 2

- 1 cup of hibiscus tea (can be consumed either cold or hot)
- 1 large green garden salad (Only 3 tablespoons of fat-free dressing, no bacon bits, no croutons. Keep it clean.)
- You can choose one of the following beverages in addition to the tea:

  1 cup of lemonade (freshly squeezed preferred)

  Unlimited plain water (flat or fizzy)

  1 cup of flavored water

  1 cup of juice (not from concentrate)

  1 cup of unsweetened iced tea

  1 cup of low-fat, reduced-fat, or fat-free milk, unsweetened soy milk, or unsweetened almond milk

SNACK 2

- 100 calories or less

MEAL 3

- 1 cup of 100-percent fresh cranberry juice (not from concentrate, no additives); mix with a little water to reduce the bitterness
- 1 chicken or turkey sandwich on 100-percent whole-wheat or 100-percent whole-grain bread; lettuce, tomato, 1 slice of cheese, and 1 teaspoon of mustard or mayo if desired (You can always substitute a medium

salad for a meal. Just remember only 3 tablespoons of fat-free dressing, no bacon bits, no croutons. Keep it clean.)

- 1 serving of veggies; it *must* come from this list:

    Broccoli

    Cauliflower

    Brussels sprouts

    Collard greens

    Kale

    Bell peppers

    Eggplants

- You can choose one of the following beverages in addition to the cranberry juice:

    1 cup of lemonade (freshly squeezed preferred)

    Unlimited plain water (flat or fizzy)

    1 cup of flavored water

    1 cup of juice (not from concentrate)

    1 cup of unsweetened iced tea

    1 cup of low-fat, reduced-fat, or fat-free milk, unsweetened soy milk, or unsweetened almond milk

MEAL 4

- Choose one item from Group A *and* one item from Group B:

    Group A

    1 small bowl of pasta with marinara sauce (*no* cream sauces)

    1 cheeseburger or hamburger (3½ inches in diameter, ½-inch thick)

    1 bowl of soup (no potatoes, no cream). Good choices are chicken noodle, vegetable, lentil,

chickpea, split pea, black bean, tomato bisque, etc. Be careful of sodium content!

5-ounce piece of turkey (no skin, no frying)

5-ounce piece of chicken (no skin, no frying)

5-ounce piece of fish (no frying)

Group B

1 serving of veggies

Small green garden salad

- Choose one of the following beverages:

1 cup of lemonade (freshly squeezed preferred)

Unlimited plain water (flat or fizzy)

1 cup of flavored water

1 cup of juice (not from concentrate)

1 cup of unsweetened iced tea

SNACK 3

- 100 calories or less

EXERCISE

- Amount of exercise today: Minimum 30 minutes. If you want to do more, all the better! Work as hard as you can!

The goal of these exercises is to push yourself to work hard in a short period of time. The time listed is how much time is expected of you to perform the exercise, not how much time you are actually present in the gym. A lot of people spend too much time in the gym not working out, but talking and all other things that have nothing to do with the real purpose of going to a gym. The clock doesn't start until you are actually moving and the clock stops when you stop. To achieve the most without wasting time it's important that you be focused and efficient. Do these exercises at moderate levels of intensity. In order for these exercises to be effective and have an impact on your calorie burn and metabolism, you really need to get your heart rate up. You don't have to go to a gym to do these exercises. You can get a tremendous workout right in your own house or backyard. Choose a workout that's different from the last one you did. Below are some 15-minute interval exercises that you should try. So if the program calls for a 45-minute workout, try 15 minutes on the treadmill, 15 minutes on the bicycle, and 15 minutes on the stair climber. It's up to you how you break it up, but note that changing your routine is typically more advantageous than doing the same exercise for the entire workout.

- Choose a combination of the items below to fulfill your exercise requirement:

  15 minutes jogging outside

  15 minutes walking/running on treadmill

  15 minutes on elliptical machine

  15 minutes on stationary or mobile bicycle

  15 minutes swimming laps

  15 minutes on stair climber

  225 jump rope revolutions

  20 minutes treadmill intervals

  15 minutes of Zumba

  15 minutes of spinning

  15 minutes of any other high-intensity cardio

  15 minutes of rowing machine

SHRED WEEK 5, DAY 2

MEAL 1

- 1 cup of lemon water. Pour 8 ounces of water, either hot or cold. Squeeze the juice from half a lemon directly into the water. Add 2 tablespoons of ground flaxseeds or flaxseed oil. Mix well and drink.
- Choose one of the following. Your choice must not exceed 250 calories.

    1 fruit smoothie

    1 Green Power Machine Smoothie (see recipe in chapter 10)

    1 veggie smoothie (You can use any veggies you want.)

- 1 piece of fruit

SNACK 1

- Choose one of the following:

    14 raw almonds

    ½ cucumber sliced with 2 tablespoons hummus

    8 baby carrots with 2 tablespoons hummus

    1 celery stalk cut into slices with 2 tablespoons hummus

MEAL 2

- 1 cup of 100-percent fresh cranberry juice (not from concentrate, no additives); mix with a little water to reduce the bitterness.

- Choose one of the following:

    3 servings of vegetables (Remember, a serving is about the size of the average person's fist.) One of the vegetables must be a dark-green leafy vegetable, such as spinach, kale, romaine lettuce, leaf lettuce, mustard greens, collard greens, chicory, or Swiss chard.

    1 large green garden salad (no croutons, no bacon bits, 4 tablespoons of fat-free or low-fat dressing)

    1 cup of brown rice or quinoa with ½ cup of beans

- You can choose one of the following beverages in addition to the cranberry juice:

    1 cup of lemonade (freshly squeezed preferred)

    Unlimited plain water (flat or fizzy)

    1 cup of flavored water

    1 cup of juice (not from concentrate)

    1 cup of unsweetened iced tea

SNACK 2

- 150 calories or less

MEAL 3

- 1 cup of hibiscus tea (can be consumed either cold or hot)
- Choose one of the following. Your choice must be different from your selection for meal 2.

    1 large green garden salad (no croutons, no bacon bits, 4 tablespoons of fat-free or low-fat dressing)

    1 fruit smoothie (200 calories or less)

    1 protein shake (200 calories or less)

- You can choose one of the following beverages in addition to the tea:

One 12-ounce can of diet soda

1 cup of lemonade (freshly squeezed preferred)

Unlimited plain water (flat or fizzy)

1 cup of flavored water

1 cup of juice (not from concentrate)

1 cup of unsweetened iced tea

SNACK 3

- Choose one of the following:

  1 apple

  1 pear

  Kale chips (see recipe in chapter 9)

  1½ cups veggie juice (not from concentrate)

  4 unsalted, gluten-free rice crackers with 3 table-spoons guacamole

MEAL 4

- Choose one of the following. Your choice must be different from your selection for meal 3.

  3 servings of vegetables (Remember, a serving is about the size of the average person's fist.)

  1 large green garden salad (no croutons, no bacon bits, 4 tablespoons of fat-free or low-fat dressing)

  1 veggie burger (3½ inches in diameter, ½-inch thick)

  1 bowl of soup (200 calories or less; no potatoes, no cream). Good choices are chicken noodle, vegetable, lentil, chickpea, split pea, black bean, tomato bisque, etc. Be careful of sodium content!

- If you choose the protein shake or soup, you should also consume 1 serving of veggies.

- Choose one of the following beverages:

    1 cup of lemonade (freshly squeezed preferred)

    Unlimited plain water (flat or fizzy)

    1 cup of flavored water

    1 cup of juice (not from concentrate)

    1 cup of unsweetened iced tea

EXERCISE

- Amount of exercise today: Minimum 45 minutes. If you want to do more, all the better! Work as hard as you can!

- Choose a combination of the items below to fulfill your exercise requirement:

    15 minutes jogging outside

    15 minutes walking/running on treadmill

    15 minutes on elliptical machine

    15 minutes on stationary or mobile bicycle

    15 minutes swimming laps

    15 minutes on stair climber

    225 jump rope revolutions

    20 minutes treadmill intervals

    15 minutes of Zumba

    15 minutes of spinning

    15 minutes of any other high-intensity cardio

    15 minutes of rowing machine

SHRED WEEK 5, DAY 3

MEAL 1

- 1 cup of lemon water. Pour 8 ounces of water, either hot or cold. Squeeze the juice from half a lemon directly into the water. Add 2 tablespoons of ground flaxseeds or flaxseed oil. Mix well and drink.
- 1 piece of fruit. This can be 1 banana, 1 apple, 1 pear, etc. It can also be ½ cup of raspberries, blueberries, blackberries, or strawberries.
- Choose one of the following. Your portion should be 1 cup cooked.
    1 small bowl of oatmeal
    1 small bowl of Cream of Wheat
    1 small bowl of grits
- 1 cup of fresh juice *not* from concentrate (grapefruit, apple, orange juice, tomato, carrot, etc.)

SNACK 1

- Choose one of the following:
    Raw trail mix (½ cup of raw nuts with sunflower or pumpkin seeds and dried fruit)
    2 dates stuffed with almonds (take out the pit and replace with a few almonds)
    ½ cup raisins, raw walnuts, and pinch of sea salt (mix together)
    3 tomato slices and fresh basil drizzled with olive oil

½ cucumber, sliced, sprinkled with pinch of sea salt and fat-free vinaigrette dressing

1 cup of unsweetened apple sauce

10 cherries mixed with handful of nuts (cashews, almonds, or walnuts)

8 baby carrots with 2 tablespoons of hummus

Ants on a log (2 celery sticks dabbed with 1 tablespoon of raw nut butter and 1 tablespoon organic raisins)

1 piece of medium-size fruit

Small beet salad

1 cup of beet juice

MEAL 2

- Choose one of the following. Your choice must be 200 calories or less.

    1 fruit smoothie

    1 protein shake

    1 bowl of soup (no potatoes, no cream). Good choices are chicken noodle, vegetable, lentil, chickpea, split pea, black bean, tomato bisque, etc. Be careful of sodium content!

- 1 piece of fruit *or* 1 serving of veggies

- Choose one of the following beverages:

    One 12-ounce can of diet soda

    1 cup of lemonade (freshly squeezed preferred)

    Unlimited plain water (flat or fizzy)

    1 cup of flavored water

    1 cup of juice (not from concentrate)

    1 cup of unsweetened iced tea

SNACK 2

- Choose one of the following:

    Raw trail mix (½ cup of raw nuts with sunflower or pumpkin seeds and dried fruit)

    2 dates stuffed with almonds (take out the pit and replace with a few almonds)

    ½ cup raisins, raw walnuts, and pinch of sea salt (mix together)

    3 tomato slices and fresh basil drizzled with olive oil

    ½ cucumber, sliced, sprinkled with pinch of sea salt and fat-free vinaigrette dressing

    1 cup of unsweetened apple sauce

    10 cherries mixed with handful of nuts (cashews, almonds, or walnuts)

    8 baby carrots with 2 tablespoons of hummus

    Ants on a log (2 celery sticks dabbed with 1 tablespoon of raw nut butter and 1 tablespoon organic raisins)

    1 piece of medium-size fruit

    Small beet salad

    1 cup of beet juice

MEAL 3

- Choose one of the following. Your choice must not exceed 250 calories. Try to choose something different from what you had in meal 2 if you can. You don't have to, but try.

    1 milk shake

    1 fruit smoothie

    1 protein shake

1 veggie shake (You can use any veggies you want.)

1 bowl of soup (no potatoes, no cream). Good choices are chicken noodle, vegetable, lentil, chickpea, split pea, black bean, tomato bisque, etc. Be careful of sodium content!

- Choose one of the following beverages. Choose a different beverage from what you chose with meal 2.

  One 12-ounce can of diet soda

  1 cup of lemonade (freshly squeezed preferred)

  Unlimited plain water (flat or fizzy)

  1 cup of flavored water

  1 cup of juice (not from concentrate)

  1 cup of unsweetened iced tea

SNACK 3

- Choose one of the following:

  Raw trail mix (½ cup of raw nuts with sunflower or pumpkin seeds and dried fruit)

  2 dates stuffed with almonds (take out the pit and replace with a few almonds)

  ½ cup raisins, raw walnuts, and pinch of sea salt (mix together)

  3 tomato slices and fresh basil drizzled with olive oil

  ½ cucumber, sliced, sprinkled with pinch of sea salt and fat-free vinaigrette dressing

  1 cup of unsweetened apple sauce

  10 cherries mixed with handful of nuts (cashews, almonds, or walnuts)

  8 baby carrots with 2 tablespoons of hummus

  Ants on a log (2 celery sticks dabbed with 1 table-

spoon of raw nut butter and 1 tablespoon organic raisins)

1 piece of medium-size fruit

Small beet salad

1 cup of beet juice

MEAL 4

- Choose from Group A *or* Group B. *Do not* choose from both.

    Group A—choose one from the following:

    5-ounce piece of chicken (no skin, no frying)

    5-ounce piece of fish (no frying)

    5-ounce piece of turkey (no skin, no frying)

    All of the above come with ½ cup of brown rice and 1 serving of veggies.

    Group B—you can have both items below:

    1 serving of lasagna (with or without meat), 4 inches × 2 inches × 1 inch

    1 serving of veggies

- Choose one of the following beverages. Choose a different beverage than what you chose with meals 2 and 3.

    1 cup of lemonade (freshly squeezed preferred)

    Unlimited plain water (flat or fizzy)

    1 cup of flavored water

    1 cup of juice (not from concentrate)

    1 cup of unsweetened iced tea

EXERCISE

- Rest Day. But if you're inspired to do something, by all means go and do it. Every minute of exercise burns more calories and gets you closer to your goal. You might even try playing a sport, which can be a fun way to burn calories without feeling like you're actually working out.

SHRED WEEK 5, DAY 4

MEAL 1

- 1 cup of lemon water. Pour 8 ounces of water, either hot or cold. Squeeze the juice from half a lemon directly into the water. Add 2 tablespoons of ground flaxseeds or flaxseed oil. Mix well and drink.
- 1 cup of raspberries, sliced strawberries, blueberries, or blackberries
- Choose one of the following. Your choice must be 200 calories or less and no sugar added.

    1 fruit smoothie

    1 protein shake

SNACK 1

- Choose one of the following:

    Raw trail mix (½ cup of raw nuts with sunflower or pumpkin seeds and dried fruit)

    2 dates stuffed with almonds (take out the pit and replace with a few almonds)

    ½ cup raisins, raw walnuts, and pinch of sea salt (mix together)

    3 tomato slices and fresh basil drizzled with olive oil

    ½ cucumber, sliced, sprinkled with pinch of sea salt and fat-free vinaigrette dressing

1 cup of unsweetened apple sauce

10 cherries mixed with handful of nuts (cashews, almonds, or walnuts)

8 baby carrots with 2 tablespoons of hummus

Ants on a log (2 celery sticks dabbed with 1 tablespoon of raw nut butter and 1 tablespoon organic raisins)

1 piece of medium-size fruit

Small beet salad

1 cup of beet juice

20 almonds

Small fruit cup

8 halves of dried apricots

2 tablespoons of sunflower seeds

4 slices of Melba whole-wheat or whole-grain toast

MEAL 2

- 1 cup of hibiscus tea (can be consumed either cold or hot)

- Choose one of the following:

    3 servings of vegetables (Remember, a serving is about the size of the average person's fist.)

    1 large green garden salad (no croutons, no bacon bits, 4 tablespoons of fat-free or low-fat dressing)

    1 protein shake (200 calories or less)

    1 bowl of soup (200 calories or less; no potatoes, no cream). Good choices are chicken noodle, vegetable, lentil, chickpea, split pea, black bean, tomato bisque, etc. Be careful of sodium content!

- If you choose the protein shake or soup, you should also consume 1 serving of veggies

- You can choose one of the following beverages in addition to the tea:

    One 12-ounce can of diet soda

    1 cup of lemonade (freshly squeezed preferred)

    Unlimited plain water (flat or fizzy)

    1 cup of flavored water

    1 cup of juice (not from concentrate)

    1 cup of unsweetened iced tea

    1 cup of low-fat, reduced-fat, or fat-free milk, unsweetened soy milk, or unsweetened almond milk

SNACK 2

- Choose one of the following:

    Raw trail mix (½ cup of raw nuts with sunflower or pumpkin seeds and dried fruit)

    2 dates stuffed with almonds (take out the pit and replace with a few almonds)

    ½ cup raisins, raw walnuts, and pinch of sea salt (mix together)

    3 tomato slices and fresh basil drizzled with olive oil

    ½ cucumber, sliced, sprinkled with pinch of sea salt and fat-free vinaigrette dressing

    1 cup of unsweetened apple sauce

    10 cherries mixed with handful of nuts (cashews, almonds, or walnuts)

    8 baby carrots with 2 tablespoons of hummus

    Ants on a log (2 celery sticks dabbed with 1 tablespoon of raw nut butter and 1 tablespoon organic raisins)

    1 piece of medium-size fruit

    Small beet salad

1 cup of beet juice

20 almonds

Small fruit cup

8 halves of dried apricots

2 tablespoons of sunflower seeds

4 slices of Melba whole-wheat or whole-grain toast

MEAL 3

- 1 cup of 100-percent fresh cranberry juice (not from concentrate, no additives); mix with a little water to reduce the bitterness

- Choose one of the following:

  1 veggie burger (3½ inches in diameter, ½-inch thick)

  5-ounce piece of lean beef (no frying)

  5-ounce piece of chicken (no skin, no frying)

  5-ounce piece of fish (no frying)

  5-ounce piece of turkey (no skin, no frying)

  1 cup of spaghetti and meatballs

  (5 ounces is about the size of a deck and a half of playing cards.)

- 1 serving of veggies

- Half of a baked sweet potato (no whipped cream or other additions; you can add 1 teaspoon of butter) or ½ cup of rice (brown preferred, but you can have white if you choose)

- You can choose one of the following beverages in addition to the cranberry juice:

  1 cup of lemonade (freshly squeezed preferred)

  Unlimited plain water (flat or fizzy)

  1 cup of flavored water

  1 cup of juice (not from concentrate)

1 cup of unsweetened iced tea

1 cup of low-fat, reduced-fat, or fat-free milk, unsweetened soy milk, or unsweetened almond milk

SNACK 3

- Choose one of the following:

Raw trail mix (½ cup of raw nuts with sunflower or pumpkin seeds and dried fruit)

2 dates stuffed with almonds (take out the pit and replace with a few almonds)

½ cup raisins, raw walnuts, and pinch of sea salt (mix together)

3 tomato slices and fresh basil drizzled with olive oil

½ cucumber, sliced, sprinkled with pinch of sea salt and fat-free vinaigrette dressing

1 cup of unsweetened apple sauce

10 cherries mixed with handful of nuts (cashews, almonds, or walnuts)

8 baby carrots with 2 tablespoons of hummus

Ants on a log (2 celery sticks dabbed with 1 tablespoon of raw nut butter and 1 tablespoon organic raisins)

1 piece of medium-size fruit

Small beet salad

1 cup of beet juice

20 almonds

Small fruit cup

8 halves of dried apricots

2 tablespoons of sunflower seeds

4 slices of Melba whole-wheat or whole-grain toast

MEAL 4

- Choose one of the following. Your choice must be 200 calories or less and no sugar added.

    1 fruit smoothie

    1 protein shake

    1 veggie smoothie

- 1 cup of beans or other legumes (no baked beans)
- Choose one of the following beverages:

    1 cup of lemonade (freshly squeezed preferred)

    Unlimited plain water (flat or fizzy)

    1 cup of flavored water

    1 cup of juice (not from concentrate)

    1 cup of unsweetened iced tea

    1 cup of low-fat, reduced-fat, or fat-free milk, unsweetened soy milk, or unsweetened almond milk

EXERCISE

- Amount of exercise today: Minimum 45 minutes. If you want to do more, all the better! Work as hard as you can!
- Choose a combination of the items below to fulfill your exercise requirement:

    15 minutes jogging outside

    15 minutes walking/running on treadmill

    15 minutes on elliptical machine

    15 minutes on stationary or mobile bicycle

    15 minutes swimming laps

    15 minutes on stair climber

    225 jump rope revolutions

    20 minutes treadmill intervals

15 minutes of Zumba

15 minutes of spinning

15 minutes of any other high-intensity cardio

15 minutes of rowing machine

SHRED WEEK 5, DAY 5

MEAL 1

- 1 cup of lemon water. Pour 8 ounce of water, either hot or cold. Squeeze the juice from half a lemon directly into the water. Add 2 tablespoons of ground flaxseeds or flaxseed oil. Mix well and drink.

- Choose from one of the following. Your choice must be 200 calories or less and no sugar added.

    1 fruit smoothie

    1 protein shake

    1 veggie shake

SNACK 1

- Choose one of the following:

    Raw trail mix (½ cup of raw nuts with sunflower or pumpkin seeds and dried fruit)

    2 dates stuffed with almonds (take out the pit and replace with a few almonds)

    ½ cup raisins, raw walnuts, and pinch of sea salt (mix together)

    3 tomato slices and fresh basil drizzled with olive oil

    ½ cucumber, sliced, sprinkled with pinch of sea salt and fat-free vinaigrette dressing

1 cup of unsweetened apple sauce

10 cherries mixed with handful of nuts (cashews, almonds, or walnuts)

8 baby carrots with 2 tablespoons of hummus

Ants on a log (2 celery sticks dabbed with 1 tablespoon of raw nut butter and 1 tablespoon organic raisins)

1 piece of medium-size fruit

Small beet salad

1 cup of beet juice

20 almonds

Small fruit cup

8 halves of dried apricots

2 tablespoons of sunflower seeds

4 slices of Melba whole-wheat or whole-grain toast

MEAL 2

- 1 cup of 100-percent fresh cranberry juice (not from concentrate, no additives); mix with a little water to reduce the bitterness
- Choose one of the following:

    2 chicken fingers

    1 cup of chicken stir-fry

    5-ounce piece of fish (no frying)

    6 jumbo shrimp (2 tablespoons cocktail sauce)

    1 cup of pasta (no cream sauce)

    3 servings of veggies

- 1 serving of veggies if you did not choose veggies above
- You can choose one of the following beverages in addition to the cranberry juice:

1 cup of lemonade (freshly squeezed preferred)

Unlimited plain water (flat or fizzy)

1 cup of flavored water

1 cup of juice (not from concentrate)

1 cup of unsweetened iced tea or 2 cups of any other kind of tea

1 cup of low-fat, reduced-fat, or fat-free milk, unsweetened soy milk, or unsweetened almond milk

SNACK 2

- Choose one of the following:

    Raw trail mix (½ cup of raw nuts with sunflower or pumpkin seeds and dried fruit)

    2 dates stuffed with almonds (take out the pit and replace with a few almonds)

    ½ cup raisins, raw walnuts, and pinch of sea salt (mix together)

    3 tomato slices and fresh basil drizzled with olive oil

    ½ cucumber, sliced, sprinkled with pinch of sea salt and fat-free vinaigrette dressing

    1 cup of unsweetened apple sauce

    10 cherries mixed with handful of nuts (cashews, almonds, or walnuts)

    8 baby carrots with 2 tablespoons of hummus

    Ants on a log (2 celery sticks dabbled with 1 tablespoon of raw nut butter and 1 tablespoon organic raisins)

    1 piece of medium-size fruit

    Small beet salad

    1 cup of beet juice

    20 almonds

Small fruit cup

8 halves of dried apricots

2 tablespoons of sunflower seeds

4 slices of Melba whole-wheat or whole-grain toast

MEAL 3

- 1 cup of hibiscus tea (can be consumed either cold or hot)
- Choose one of the following. Your choice must be 200 calories or less and no sugar added.

    1 fruit smoothie

    1 protein shake

    1 veggie shake

- 1 serving of veggies
- You can choose one of the following beverages in addition to the tea:

    1 cup of lemonade (freshly squeezed preferred)

    Unlimited plain water (flat or fizzy)

    1 cup of flavored water

    1 cup of juice (not from concentrate)

    1 cup of unsweetened iced tea or 2 cups of any other kind of tea

    1 cup of low-fat, reduced-fat, or fat-free milk, unsweetened soy milk, or unsweetened almond milk

SNACK 3

- Choose one of the following:

    Raw trail mix (½ cup of raw nuts with sunflower or pumpkin seeds and dried fruit)

    2 dates stuffed with almonds (take out the pit and replace with a few almonds)

½ cup raisins, raw walnuts, and pinch of sea salt (mix together)

3 tomato slices and fresh basil drizzled with olive oil

½ cucumber, sliced, sprinkled with pinch of sea salt and fat-free vinaigrette dressing

1 cup of unsweetened apple sauce

10 cherries mixed with handful of nuts (cashews, almonds, or walnuts)

8 baby carrots with 2 tablespoons of hummus

Ants on a log (2 celery sticks dabbed with 1 tablespoon of raw nut butter and 1 tablespoon organic raisins)

1 piece of medium-size fruit

Small beet salad

1 cup of beet juice

20 almonds

Small fruit cup

8 halves of dried apricots

2 tablespoons of sunflower seeds

4 slices of Melba whole-wheat or whole-grain toast

MEAL 4

- Choose one of the following:

    5-ounce piece of lean beef (no frying)

    5-ounce piece of chicken (no skin, no frying)

    5-ounce piece of fish (no frying)

    5-ounce piece of turkey (no skin, no frying)

    1 cup of spaghetti and meatballs

    (5 ounces is about the size of a deck and a half of playing cards.)

- 1 serving of veggies
- Half of a baked sweet potato (no whipped cream or other additions; you can add 1 teaspoon of butter) *or* ½ cup of rice (brown preferred, but you can have white if you choose)
- Choose one of the following beverages:

    1 cup of lemonade (freshly squeezed preferred)

    Unlimited plain water (flat or fizzy)

    1 cup of flavored water

    1 cup of juice (not from concentrate)

    1 cup of unsweetened iced tea or 2 cups of any other kind of tea

    1 cup of low-fat, reduced-fat, or fat-free milk, unsweetened soy milk, or unsweetened almond milk

SNACK 4

- Choose one of the following:

    Raw trail mix (½ cup of raw nuts with sunflower or pumpkin seeds and dried fruit)

    2 dates stuffed with almonds (take out the pit and replace with a few almonds)

    ½ cup raisins, raw walnuts, and pinch of sea salt (mix together)

    3 tomato slices and fresh basil drizzled with olive oil

    ½ cucumber, sliced, sprinkled with pinch of sea salt and fat-free vinaigrette dressing

    1 cup of unsweetened apple sauce

    10 cherries mixed with handful of nuts (cashews, almonds, or walnuts)

    8 baby carrots with 2 tablespoons of hummus

Ants on a log (2 celery sticks dabbed with 1 tablespoon of raw nut butter and 1 tablespoon organic raisins)

1 piece of medium-size fruit

Small beet salad

1 cup of beet juice

20 almonds

Small fruit cup

8 halves of dried apricots

2 tablespoons of sunflower seeds

4 slices of Melba whole-wheat or whole-grain toast

EXERCISE

- Amount of exercise today: Minimum 45 minutes. If you want to do more, all the better! Work as hard as you can!

- Choose a combination of the items below to fulfill your exercise requirement:

    15 minutes jogging outside

    15 minutes walking/running on treadmill

    15 minutes on elliptical machine

    15 minutes on stationary or mobile bicycle

    15 minutes swimming laps

    15 minutes on stair climber

    225 jump rope revolutions

    20 minutes treadmill intervals

    15 minutes of Zumba

    15 minutes of spinning

    15 minutes of any other high-intensity cardio

    15 minutes of rowing machine

SHRED WEEK 5, DAY 6

MEAL 1

- 1 cup of lemon water. Pour 8 ounces of water, either hot or cold. Squeeze the juice from half a lemon directly into the water. Add 2 tablespoons of ground flaxseeds or flaxseed oil. Mix well and drink.
- 1 piece of fruit
- Choose one of the following:

    1 small bowl of oatmeal (1 ½ cups cooked)

    2 egg whites *or* 1 egg-white omelet with diced veggies (made with 2 egg whites max)

    1 small bowl of sugar-free cereal with fat-free, skim, or 1-percent fat milk

    1 grilled cheese sandwich on 100-percent whole-grain or 100-percent whole-wheat bread

- 1 cup of fresh juice *not* from concentrate (grapefruit, apple, orange juice, tomato, carrot, etc.)

SNACK 1

- Choose one of the following:

    Raw trail mix (½ cup of raw nuts with sunflower or pumpkin seeds and dried fruit)

    2 dates stuffed with almonds (take out the pit and replace with a few almonds)

    ½ cup raisins, raw walnuts, and pinch of sea salt (mix together)

    3 tomato slices and fresh basil drizzled with olive oil

½ cucumber, sliced, sprinkled with pinch of sea salt and fat-free vinaigrette dressing

1 cup of unsweetened apple sauce

10 cherries mixed with handful of nuts (cashews, almonds, or walnuts)

8 baby carrots with 2 tablespoons of hummus

Ants on a log (2 celery sticks dabbed with 1 tablespoon of raw nut butter and 1 tablespoon organic raisins)

1 piece of medium-size fruit

Small beet salad

1 cup of beet juice

20 almonds

Small fruit cup

8 halves of dried apricots

2 tablespoons of sunflower seeds

4 slices of Melba whole-wheat or whole-grain toast

MEAL 2

- 1 cup of hibiscus tea (can be consumed either cold or hot)

- Choose one of the following. Your choice must be 250 calories or less.

    1 fruit smoothie

    1 protein shake

    1 veggie shake

    1 bowl of soup (no potatoes, no cream, no meat). Good choices are vegetable, lentil, chickpea, split pea, black bean, tomato bisque, etc. Be careful of sodium content!

- 1 piece of fruit *or* 1 serving of veggies

- Choose one of the following beverages in addition to the tea:

    1 cup of lemonade (freshly squeezed preferred)

    Unlimited plain water (flat or fizzy)

    1 cup of flavored water

    1 cup of juice (not from concentrate)

    1 cup of unsweetened iced tea or 2 cups of any other kind of tea

    1 cup of low-fat, reduced-fat, or fat-free milk, unsweetened soy milk, or unsweetened almond milk

SNACK 2

- Choose one from the following.

    Raw trail mix (½ cup of raw nuts with sunflower or pumpkin seeds and dried fruit)

    2 dates stuffed with almonds (take out the pit and replace with a few almonds)

    ½ cup raisins, raw walnuts, and pinch of sea salt (mix together)

    3 tomato slices and fresh basil drizzled with olive oil

    ½ cucumber, sliced, sprinkled with pinch of sea salt and fat-free vinaigrette dressing

    1 cup of unsweetened apple sauce

    10 cherries mixed with handful of nuts (cashews, almonds, or walnuts)

    8 baby carrots with 2 tablespoons of hummus

    Ants on a log (2 celery sticks dabbed with 1 tablespoon of raw nut butter and 1 tablespoon organic raisins)

    1 piece of medium-size fruit

    Small beet salad

1 cup of beet juice

20 almonds

Small fruit cup

8 halves of dried apricots

2 tablespoons of sunflower seeds

4 slices of Melba whole-wheat or whole-grain toast

MEAL 3

- 1 cup of 100-percent fresh cranberry juice (not from concentrate, no additives); mix with a little water to reduce the bitterness
- Choose one of the following. Your choice must be 200 calories or less. Try to choose something different from what you chose for meal 2.

  1 fruit smoothie

  1 protein shake

  1 bowl of soup (no potatoes, no cream). Good choices are vegetable, lentil, chickpea, split pea, black bean, tomato bisque, etc. Be careful of sodium (salt) content!

- 1 piece of fruit *or* 1 serving of veggies
- Choose one of the following beverages in addition to the cranberry juice:

  1 cup of lemonade (freshly squeezed preferred)

  Unlimited plain water (flat or fizzy)

  1 cup of flavored water

  1 cup of juice (not from concentrate)

  1 cup of unsweetened iced tea or 2 cups of any other kind of tea

  1 cup of low-fat, reduced-fat, or fat-free milk, unsweetened soy milk, or unsweetened almond milk

SNACK 3

- Choose one of the following:

    Raw trail mix (½ cup of raw nuts with sunflower or pumpkin seeds and dried fruit)

    2 dates stuffed with almonds (take out the pit and replace with a few almonds)

    ½ cup raisins, raw walnuts, and pinch of sea salt (mix together)

    3 tomato slices and fresh basil drizzled with olive oil

    ½ cucumber, sliced, sprinkled with pinch of sea salt and fat-free vinaigrette dressing

    1 cup of unsweetened apple sauce

    10 cherries mixed with handful of nuts (cashews, almonds, or walnuts)

    8 baby carrots with 2 tablespoons of hummus

    Ants on a log (2 celery sticks dabbed with 1 tablespoon of raw nut butter and 1 tablespoon organic raisins)

    1 piece of medium-size fruit

    Small beet salad

    1 cup of beet juice

    20 almonds

    Small fruit cup

    8 halves of dried apricots

    2 tablespoons of sunflower seeds

    4 slices of Melba whole-wheat or whole-grain toast

MEAL 4

- 1 cup of beans (no baked beans)
- Choose one of the following. Your choice must be

200 calories or less. Try to choose something different from what you chose for meal 3.

1 fruit smoothie

1 protein shake

1 veggie shake

- You can choose one of the following beverages in addition to the tea:

    1 cup of lemonade (freshly squeezed preferred)

    Unlimited plain water (flat or fizzy)

    1 cup of flavored water

    1 cup of juice (not from concentrate)

    1 cup of unsweetened iced tea or 2 cups of any other kind of tea

    1 cup of low-fat, reduced-fat, or fat-free milk, unsweetened soy milk, or unsweetened almond milk

SNACK 4

- Choose one of the following.

    Raw trail mix (½ cup of raw nuts with sunflower or pumpkin seeds and dried fruit)

    2 dates stuffed with almonds (take out the pit and replace with a few almonds)

    ½ cup raisins, raw walnuts, and pinch of sea salt (mix together)

    3 tomato slices and fresh basil drizzled with olive oil

    ½ cucumber, sliced, sprinkled with pinch of sea salt and fat-free vinaigrette dressing

    1 cup of unsweetened apple sauce

    10 cherries mixed with handful of nuts (cashews, almonds, or walnuts)

    8 baby carrots with 2 tablespoons of hummus

Ants on a log (2 celery sticks dabbed with 1 tablespoon of raw nut butter and 1 tablespoon organic
raisins)

1 piece of medium-size fruit

Small beet salad

1 cup of beet juice

20 almonds

Small fruit cup

8 halves of dried apricots

2 tablespoons of sunflower seeds

4 slices of Melba whole-wheat or whole-grain toast

EXERCISE

- Rest Day. But if you're inspired to do something, by
  all means go and do it. Every minute of exercise burns
  more calories and gets you closer to your goal. You
  might even try playing a sport, which can be a fun way
  to burn calories without feeling like you're actually
  working out.

SHRED WEEK 5, DAY 7

MEAL 1

- 1 cup of lemon water. Pour 8 ounces of water, either
  hot or cold. Squeeze the juice from half a lemon directly into the water. Add 2 tablespoons of ground
  flaxseeds or flaxseed oil. Mix well and drink.

- Choose one of the following. Your choice must be 200
  calories or less.

1 fruit smoothie

1 protein shake

1 veggie shake

- 1 piece of fruit

SNACK 1

- Choose one of the following:

    Raw trail mix (½ cup of raw nuts with sunflower or pumpkin seeds and dried fruit)

    2 dates stuffed with almonds (take out the pit and replace with a few almonds)

    ½ cup raisins, raw walnuts, and pinch of sea salt (mix together)

    3 tomato slices and fresh basil drizzled with olive oil

    ½ cucumber, sliced, sprinkled with pinch of sea salt and fat-free vinaigrette dressing

    1 cup of unsweetened apple sauce

    10 cherries mixed with handful of nuts (cashews, almonds, or walnuts)

    8 baby carrots with 2 tablespoons of hummus

    Ants on a log (2 celery sticks dabbed with 1 tablespoon of raw nut butter and 1 tablespoon organic raisins)

    1 piece of medium-size fruit

    Small beet salad

    1 cup of beet juice

    20 almonds

    Small fruit cup

    8 halves of dried apricots

    2 tablespoons of sunflower seeds

    4 slices of Melba whole-wheat or whole-grain toast

MEAL 2

- 1 cup of 100-percent fresh cranberry juice (not from concentrate, no additives); mix with a little water to reduce the bitterness
- Choose one of the following. Your choice must be 250 calories or less.

    1 protein shake

    1 veggie shake

    1 bowl of soup (no potatoes, no cream, no meat). Good choices are vegetable, lentil, chickpea, split pea, black bean, tomato bisque, etc. Be careful of sodium content!

- You can choose one of the following beverages in addition to the cranberry juice:

    1 cup of lemonade (freshly squeezed preferred)

    Unlimited plain water (flat or fizzy)

    1 cup of flavored water

    1 cup of juice (not from concentrate)

    1 cup of unsweetened iced tea

    1 cup of low-fat, reduced-fat, or fat-free milk, unsweetened soy milk, or unsweetened almond milk

SNACK 2

- Choose one of the following:

    Raw trail mix (½ cup of raw nuts with sunflower or pumpkin seeds and dried fruit)

    2 dates stuffed with almonds (take out the pit and replace with a few almonds)

    ½ cup raisins, raw walnuts, and pinch of sea salt (mix together)

    3 tomato slices and fresh basil drizzled with olive oil

½ cucumber, sliced, sprinkled with pinch of sea salt and fat-free vinaigrette dressing

1 cup of unsweetened apple sauce

10 cherries mixed with handful of nuts (cashews, almonds, or walnuts)

8 baby carrots with 2 tablespoons of hummus

Ants on a log (2 celery sticks dabbed with 1 tablespoon of raw nut butter and 1 tablespoon organic raisins)

1 piece of medium-size fruit

Small beet salad

1 cup of beet juice

20 almonds

Small fruit cup

8 halves of dried apricots

2 tablespoons of sunflower seeds

4 slices of Melba whole-wheat or whole-grain toast

MEAL 3

- 1 cup of hibiscus tea (can be consumed either cold or hot)

- Choose from Group A *or* Group B. *Do not* choose from both.

    Group A—choose one from the following:

        5-ounce piece of chicken (no skin, no frying)

        5-ounce piece of fish (no frying)

        5-ounce piece of turkey (no skin, no frying)

    All of the above come with ½ cup of brown rice and 1 serving of veggies.

Group B—you can have both items below:

1 serving of lasagna (with or without meat), 4 inches × 2 inches × 1 inch

1 serving of veggies

- You can choose one of the following beverages in addition to the tea:

1 cup of lemonade (freshly squeezed preferred)

Unlimited plain water (flat or fizzy)

1 cup of flavored water

1 cup of juice (not from concentrate)

1 cup of unsweetened iced tea

1 cup of low-fat, reduced-fat, or fat-free milk, unsweetened soy milk, or unsweetened almond milk

SNACK 3

- Choose one of the following:

Raw trail mix (½ cup of raw nuts with sunflower or pumpkin seeds and dried fruit)

2 dates stuffed with almonds (take out the pit and replace with a few almonds)

½ cup raisins, raw walnuts, and pinch of sea salt (mix together)

3 tomato slices and fresh basil drizzled with olive oil

½ cucumber, sliced, sprinkled with pinch of sea salt and fat-free vinaigrette dressing

1 cup of unsweetened apple sauce

10 cherries mixed with handful of nuts (cashews, almonds, or walnuts)

8 baby carrots with 2 tablespoons of hummus

Ants on a log (2 celery sticks dabbed with 1 tablespoon of raw nut butter and 1 tablespoon organic
raisins)

1 piece of medium-size fruit

Small beet salad

1 cup of beet juice

20 almonds

Small fruit cup

8 halves of dried apricots

2 tablespoons of sunflower seeds

4 slices of Melba whole-wheat or whole-grain toast

MEAL 4

- Choose one of the following. Your choice must be 200
calories or less.

    1 fruit smoothie

    1 protein shake

    1 bowl of soup (no potatoes, no cream). Good choices
    are chicken noodle, vegetable, lentil, chickpea,
    split pea, black bean, tomato bisque, etc. Be careful
    of sodium content!

- 1 serving of veggies
- ½ cup of brown rice (white rice allowed also)
- You can choose one of the following beverages:

    1 cup of lemonade (freshly squeezed preferred)

    Unlimited plain water (flat or fizzy)

    1 cup of flavored water

    1 cup of juice (not from concentrate)

    1 cup of unsweetened iced tea or 2 cups of any other
    kind of tea

1 cup of low-fat, reduced-fat, or fat-free milk, unsweetened soy milk, or unsweetened almond milk

EXERCISE

- Amount of exercise today: Minimum 45 minutes. Break this up into two workouts. The first workout must happen before 12:00 P.M. The second workout must happen after 2:00 P.M.
- Choose a combination of the items below to fulfill your exercise requirement:

   15 minutes jogging outside

   15 minutes walking/running on treadmill

   15 minutes on elliptical machine

   15 minutes on stationary or mobile bicycle

   15 minutes swimming laps

   15 minutes on stair climber

   225 jump rope revolutions

   20 minutes treadmill intervals

   15 minutes of Zumba

   15 minutes of spinning

   15 minutes of any other high-intensity cardio

   15 minutes of rowing machine

CHAPTER 8

Week 6: Explode

Quietly stand in front of the mirror, and look deeply into your eyes as if you're trying to see all the way into the depths of your soul. You have done it! Starting from that moment when you looked at the first pages of Prime, doubting whether you could really do the program and speculating if the plan would really help you lose weight, and now here you stand, preparing to embark on the final leg of your six-week journey. You have lost weight, your energy levels are at a peak, and you've gained a confidence in yourself and in your abilities to stay focused and determined. Now you are ready to Explode and reach even greater heights of success.

Regardless of how much weight you have lost so far, the fact that you've made it to this week means that you have succeeded. SHRED is designed for you to lose weight in a consistent manner, not all at once. Your body and mind are much different from what they were just five weeks ago. You need to acknowledge your growth and embrace the new you. SHREDDING is not just about taking off the excess weight, but also about SHREDDING some of the mental stumbling blocks and obstacles that impeded your progress in the past. Your body has shed fat as well as increased your muscle tone, something critical to increasing your metabolism. Now it's time to put it all together and continue to make progress.

As with the other weeks, you need to continue to burn more calories. Don't take your foot off the gas pedal because you perceive yourself as coasting downhill. The harder you work, the better the results, the closer you will be to your goal. Before you start this week, take a few minutes to reflect on the past five weeks. There were plenty of times you didn't think you'd make it, or you were frustrated that you couldn't have your favorite food. You've been through all types of emotions and here you are standing all the better for it, lighter and more energetic. It's normal to have thoughts or urges to return to bad habits or make poor choices. No one is perfect, and I never expect or ask for perfection. But when you feel tired or vulnerable, close your eyes and softly repeat this mantra: "I will not give back all that I have worked so hard to earn. I can and must do this. It's in my control!"

This may be the last "official" week you SHRED if you have reached your goal. Or this may mean the end of just the first cycle as there are other cycles you will complete to reach your goal. Remember that the best weight loss is a gradual process. You didn't put on all of this extra weight in six weeks—or even six months—so it's unrealistic and unfair to ask yourself to try to lose it all in such a short period of time. You must not forget that it's much easier to gain weight than it is to lose it, so cut yourself some slack. This week you will have fun—each day is designed to be different from the next. The variety in the types and quantity of food and beverages keeps you moving along from one day to the next. Use all of the knowledge you've acquired and all of the skills you've developed these last five weeks and *Explode* into the rest of your new life. Believe! Work hard! Have fun!

SHRED WEEK 6 GUIDELINES

▶ Weigh yourself in the morning before starting the program and record it. Don't weigh yourself throughout the week. Your next weigh-in will be the same day the following week in the morning. Weigh yourself in the same manner as you did in the beginning. If you weighed in without wearing clothes initially, then do that again. If you weighed in wearing certain clothes, wear the same clothes for the second weigh-in. Use the same scale both times. *Don't* use a different scale as scales can differ by several pounds.

▶ You must eat something every 3 to 4 hours even if you're not hungry, but *don't* stuff yourself. Eat until you're no longer hungry, but *don't eat until you're full*. If you need less than what's recommended, then great, go ahead and eat less, which is even better. Switching meals is permitted, but try to switch as infrequently as possible. For example, if you know that what's listed for meal 3 is easier to get than what's listed for meal 2, then go ahead and switch them. Looking at the day's meals in advance is important as it allows you to best prepare for what's ahead.

▶ Five of the seven days you must do some type of

cardiovascular exercise, commonly called cardio. Pay attention to the guidelines written for that day. If you need to exercise on different days than listed, then go ahead and do that as long as you get five days of cardio-related physical activity in a seven-day period.

▶ If you don't eat meat, make the substitutions appropriately with fish or vegetables.

▶ This week, all shakes and smoothies have different calorie guidelines, so pay attention. Avoid added sugars if possible in those items that you buy in the store.

▶ When cooking or buying your soups, still make sure you're following the guidelines as written for that meal. Because the days are different, you need to keep checking the calories as they will vary from one day to the next. Make sure the soup is low in sodium (salt); this means the sodium or Na+ line on the label should say no more than 480 milligrams per serving. Try eating things made with sea salt as it still gives you the flavor but has less sodium content.

NEW THIS WEEK

1. Because each day is meant to be different, be careful to read through the menu first and make sure you are prepared for what you'll need.

2. There are two days where you are expected to have two exercise sessions. Please stay true to that schedule.

3. You are not allowed to have the same meal/shake/smoothie more than once in a day, so make your choices accordingly.

4. Alcohol is allowed this week, but please be careful to consume as suggested. Don't overindulge these liquid calories that return little in the way of nutrition and weight loss.

▶ Soups can be consumed with 2 saltine crackers if desired.

▶ The liquid meals must be eaten with either 1 piece of fruit *or* 1 serving of vegetables.

▶ You must consume 1 cup of water before eating a meal; you must consume 1 cup of water during your meal. You can add lemon or lime to your water and you can drink fizzy water if you desire.

▶ You are allowed to drink coffee, but only 1 small cup per day. Stay away from all of those fancy coffee preparations that have a lot of calories. Your coffee should contain no more than 50 calories

▶ Do not eat the last meal within 90 minutes of going to sleep.

▶ You can eat a 100-calorie snack before going to bed if desired.

▶ Be smart in your snack choices. Avoid chips and doughnuts and candy; you can have them some of the time, but don't eat them often. If you must have something like these items, make it only one of your snacks for the day and use healthier options for the other snacks.

▶ You don't have to eat all of the food on the day's menu if you don't want to, but no skipping meals, no doubling up on meals, and no exceeding the meal guidelines in size and volume.

▶ Condiments such as ketchup, mayo, and mustard are allowed, but no more than a teaspoon at each meal. The same goes for soy sauce.

▶ Spices are unlimited.

▶ While fresh fruit is always preferred, canned and frozen fruit are allowed. Just make sure they are water-based and there are no added sugars.

▶ Canned and frozen vegetables are allowed. Please be aware of the sodium content.

▶ As far as beverages are concerned, you are allowed as much water as you like per day. Here are some other beverage guidelines:

No regular soda
One 12-ounce can of diet soda allowed each day
Flavored waters allowed, but keep them under 60 calories
1 bottle of sports drink allowed per day, but keep it under 60 calories
For alcohol, 1 mixed drink allowed twice a week, *or* 3 light beers allowed per week, *or* 3 regular glasses of wine (red or white) allowed per week

Timing is critical to the success of this plan. It might be difficult at first, but plan in advance and do the best you can. Skipping meals is not advised. Even if you eat just a small portion, try to eat something on schedule. A sample day's schedule during Explode might look something like the grid below, but for each and every day, the order of the meals and snacks is both intended and critical. And on some days, there's a bonus fourth snack, so follow each day's directions carefully.

8:30 A.M.	10:00 A.M.	11:30 A.M.	1:00 P.M.	3:30 P.M.	7:00 P.M.	8:30 P.M.
Meal 1	Snack 1	Meal 2	Snack 2	Meal 3	Meal 4	Snack 3

SHRED WEEK 6, DAY 1

- 3 slices of 100-percent whole-grain or 100-percent whole-wheat bread can be consumed at any point throughout the day at any time; however, *only 3* slices.

MEAL 1

- 1 piece of fruit
- Choose one of the following:

    1 small bowl of oatmeal (1½ cups cooked)

    2 egg whites *or* 1 egg-white omelet with diced veggies (made with 2 egg whites max)

    1 small bowl of sugar-free cereal with fat-free, skim, or 1-percent fat milk

    1 container of low-fat or fat-free yogurt

- 1 cup of fresh juice *not* from concentrate (grapefruit, apple, orange juice, tomato, carrot, etc.)

SNACK 1
- 100 calories or less

MEAL 2
- Choose one of the following. Your choice must not exceed 200 calories and must not have any added sugars.
  1 fruit smoothie
  1 protein shake
  1 bowl of soup (no potatoes, no cream)
- 1 piece of fruit *or* 1 serving of veggies

SNACK 2
- 150 calories or less

MEAL 3
- 1 small green garden salad (no bacon bits, no croutons, 3 tablespoons fat-free dressing only)
- Choose one of the following:
  4–6-ounce piece of chicken (no skin, no frying)
  4–6-ounce piece of turkey (no skin, no frying)
  4–6-ounce piece of fish (no frying)
  You can have 1 slice of cheese if desired.
- 1 serving of veggies

MEAL 4
- 3 servings of veggies (make sure one serving of the veggies is dark green and leafy)
- 1 cup of beans or other legumes (no baked beans)

SNACK 3
- 100 calories or less

EXERCISE

- Amount of exercise today: Minimum 30 minutes. If you want to do more, all the better! Work as hard as you can!

The goal of these exercises is to push yourself to work hard in a short period of time. The time listed is how much time is expected of you to perform the exercise, not how much time you are actually present in the gym. A lot of people spend too much time in the gym not working out, but talking and doing all other things that have nothing to do with the real purpose of going to a gym. The clock doesn't start until you are actually moving and the clock stops when you stop. To achieve the most without wasting time it's important that you be focused and efficient. Do these exercises at moderate levels of intensity. In order for these to be effective and have an impact on your calorie burn and metabolism, you really need to get your heart rate up. You don't have to go to a gym to do these exercises. You can get a tremendous workout right in your own house or backyard. Try to choose a workout that's different from the last one you did. Below are some 15-minute interval exercises that you should try. So if the program calls for a 45-minute workout, try 15 minutes on the treadmill, 15 minutes on the bicycle, and 15 minutes on the stair climber. It's up to you how you break it up, but note that changing your routine is typically more advantageous than doing the same exercise for the entire workout.

- Choose a combination of the items below to fulfill your exercise requirement:

    15 minutes jogging outside

    15 minutes walking/running on treadmill

    15 minutes on elliptical machine

    15 minutes on stationary or mobile bicycle

    15 minutes swimming laps

    15 minutes on stair climber

    225 jump rope revolutions

    20 minutes treadmill intervals

    15 minutes of Zumba

    15 minutes of spinning

    15 minutes of any other high-intensity cardio

    15 minutes of rowing machine

SHRED WEEK 6, DAY 2

MEAL 1

- Choose one of the following. Your choice must be 200 calories or less.

    1 fruit smoothie

    1 protein shake

    1 veggie shake

    One 6-ounce container of low-fat yogurt

- 1 piece of fruit

SNACK 1

- 150 calories or less

MEAL 2

- 1 cup of lemon water. Pour 8 ounces of water, either hot or cold. Squeeze the juice from half a lemon directly into the water. If you like, add ½ teaspoon of sugar. Mix well and drink.
- 1 chicken or turkey sandwich on 100-percent whole-wheat or 100-percent whole-grain bread; lettuce, tomato, 1 slice of cheese, and 1 teaspoon of mustard or mayo if desired
- 1 small green garden salad (Only 3 tablespoons of fat-free dressing, no bacon bits, no croutons. Keep it clean.)

SNACK 2

- 100 calories or less

MEAL 3

- Choose one of the following. Your choice must be 200 calories or less.

  1 fruit smoothie

  1 protein shake

  1 veggie shake

  1 bowl of soup (no potatoes, no cream). Good choices are chicken noodle, vegetable, lentil, chickpea, split pea, black bean, tomato bisque, etc. Be careful of sodium content!
- 1 piece of fruit *or* 1 serving of veggies

SNACK 3

- 100 calories or less

MEAL 4

- Choose one of the following:

    5-ounce piece of chicken (no skin, no frying)

    5-ounce piece of fish (no frying)

    5-ounce piece of turkey (no skin, no frying)

    (5 ounces is about the size of a deck and a half of playing cards.)

- 1 serving of veggies
- ½ cup of cooked brown or white rice

EXERCISE

- Amount of exercise today: Minimum 45 minutes. Break this up into two sessions. The first session must be done before 12:00 P.M. The second session can be done anytime after 2:00 P.M. If you want to do more, all the better! Work as hard as you can!
- Choose a combination of the items below to fulfill your exercise requirement:

    15 minutes jogging outside

    15 minutes walking/running on treadmill

    15 minutes on elliptical machine

    15 minutes on stationary or mobile bicycle

    15 minutes swimming laps

    15 minutes on stair climber

    225 jump rope revolutions

    20 minutes treadmill intervals

    15 minutes of Zumba

    15 minutes of spinning

    15 minutes of any other high-intensity cardio

    15 minutes of rowing machine

SHRED WEEK 6, DAY 3

MEAL 1

- 1 cup of lemon water. Pour 8 ounces of water, either hot or cold. Squeeze the juice from half a lemon directly into the water. If you like, add ½ teaspoon of sugar. Mix well and drink.
- Choose one of the following. Your choice must be 200 calories or less.

    1 fruit smoothie

    1 protein shake

    1 veggie shake

- 1 piece of fruit

SNACK 1

- 100 calories or less

MEAL 2

- Choose one of the following:

    1 protein shake

    1 veggie shake

    1 bowl of soup (no potatoes, no cream, no meat). Good choices are vegetable, lentil, chickpea, split pea, black bean, tomato bisque, etc. Be careful of sodium content!

SNACK 2

- 150 calories or less

MEAL 3

- Choose from Group A *or* Group B. *Do not* choose from both.

    Group A—choose one of the following:

    5-ounce piece of chicken (no skin, no frying)

    5-ounce piece of fish (no frying)

    5-ounce piece of turkey (no skin, no frying)

    All of the above come with ½ cup of cooked brown rice and 1 serving of veggies.

    Group B—you can have both items below:

    1 serving of lasagna (with or without meat), 4 inches × 2 inches × 1 inch

    1 serving of veggies

MEAL 4

- Choose one of the following. Your choice must be 200 calories or less.

    1 fruit smoothie

    1 protein shake

    1 bowl of soup (no potatoes, no cream). Good choices are chicken noodle, vegetable, lentil, chickpea, split pea, black bean, tomato bisque, etc. Be careful of sodium content!

SNACK 3

- 100 calories or less

EXERCISE

- Rest Day. But if you're inspired to do something, by all means go and do it. Every minute of exercise burns more calories and gets you closer to your goal. You might even try playing a sport, which can be a fun way to burn calories without feeling like you're actually working out.

SHRED WEEK 6, DAY 4

MEAL 1

- 1 cup of lemon water. Pour 8 ounces of water, either hot or cold. Squeeze the juice from half a lemon directly into the water. If you like, add ½ teaspoon of sugar. Mix well and drink.
- 1 piece of fruit. This can be 1 banana, 1 apple, 1 pear, etc. It can also be ½ cup of raspberries, blueberries, blackberries, or strawberries.
- Choose one of the following:
    1 small bowl of oatmeal (1 ½ cups cooked)
    2 egg whites *or* 1 egg-white omelet with diced veggies (made with 2 egg whites max)
    1 small bowl of sugar-free cereal with fat-free, skim, or 1-percent fat milk
- ½ cup of fresh juice *not* from concentrate (grapefruit, apple, orange juice, tomato, carrot, etc.)

SNACK 1

- 100 calories or less

MEAL 2

- 1 chicken or turkey sandwich on 100-percent whole-wheat or 100-percent whole-grain bread; lettuce, to-

mato, 1 slice of cheese, and 1 teaspoon of mustard or mayo if desired
- 1 small green garden salad (Only 3 tablespoons of fat-free dressing, no bacon bits, no croutons. Keep it clean.)
- Choose one of the following beverages:

  One 12-ounce can of diet soda

  1 cup of lemonade (freshly squeezed preferred)

  Unlimited plain water (flat or fizzy)

  1 cup of flavored water

  1 cup of juice (not from concentrate)

  1 cup of unsweetened iced tea

  1 cup of low-fat, reduced-fat, or fat-free milk, unsweetened soy milk, or unsweetened almond milk

SNACK 2

- 100 calories or less

MEAL 3

- Choose one of the following. Your choice must not exceed 200 calories. Try to choose something different from what you had in meal 2 if you can. You don't have to, but try.

  1 milk shake

  1 fruit smoothie

  1 protein shake

  1 veggie shake (You can use any veggies you want.)

  1 bowl of soup (no potatoes, no cream). Good choices are chicken noodle, vegetable, lentil, chickpea, split pea, black bean, tomato bisque, etc. Be careful of sodium content!

- Choose one of the following beverages. Choose a different beverage from what you chose for meal 2.

    One 12-ounce can of diet soda

    1 cup of lemonade (freshly squeezed preferred)

    Unlimited plain water (flat or fizzy)

    1 cup of flavored water

    1 cup of juice (not from concentrate)

    1 cup of unsweetened iced tea

MEAL 4

- Choose one item from Group A *and* one item from Group B

    Group A

    1 small bowl of pasta with marinara sauce (*no* cream sauces)

    2 small-to-medium slices of pizza (triangular cut: 4 inches width across crust, 6 inches in length)

    1 cheeseburger or hamburger (3½ inches in diameter, ½-inch thick)

    1 bowl of soup (no potatoes, no cream). Good choices are chicken noodle, vegetable, lentil, chickpea, split pea, black bean, tomato bisque, etc. Be careful of sodium content!

    5-ounce piece of turkey (no skin, no frying)

    5-ounce piece of chicken (no skin, no frying)

    5-ounce piece of fish (no frying)

    Group B

    French fries (about 12 skinny fries or 6 steak fries)

    1 serving of veggies

    Small green garden salad

- Choose one of the following beverages. Choose a

different beverage from what you chose for meals 2 and 3.

    One 12-ounce can of diet soda

    1 cup of lemonade (freshly squeezed preferred)

    Unlimited plain water (flat or fizzy)

    1 cup of flavored water

    1 cup of juice (not from concentrate)

    1 cup of unsweetened iced tea

SNACK 3

- 100 calories or less

EXERCISE

- Amount of exercise today: Minimum 45 minutes. If you want to do more, all the better! Work as hard as you can!
- Choose a combination of the items below to fulfill your exercise requirement:

    15 minutes jogging outside

    15 minutes walking/running on treadmill

    15 minutes on elliptical machine

    15 minutes on stationary or mobile bicycle

    15 minutes swimming laps

    15 minutes on stair climber

    225 jump rope revolutions

    20 minutes treadmill intervals

    15 minutes of Zumba

    15 minutes of spinning

    15 minutes of any other high-intensity cardio

    15 minutes of rowing machine

SHRED WEEK 6, DAY 5

MEAL 1

- 1 cup of lemon water. Pour 8 ounces of water, either hot or cold. Squeeze the juice from half a lemon directly into the water. Add 2 tablespoons of ground flaxseeds or flaxseed oil. Mix well and drink.
- 1 cup of raspberries, sliced strawberries, blueberries, or blackberries
- Choose one of the following. Your choice must be 200 calories or less and no sugar added.

    1 fruit smoothie

    1 protein shake

SNACK 1

- Choose one of the following:

    Raw trail mix (½ cup of raw nuts with sunflower or pumpkin seeds and dried fruit)

    2 dates stuffed with almonds (take out the pit and replace with a few almonds)

    ½ cup raisins, raw walnuts, and pinch of sea salt (mix together)

    3 tomato slices and fresh basil drizzled with olive oil

    ½ cucumber, sliced, sprinkled with pinch of sea salt and fat-free vinaigrette dressing

    1 cup of unsweetened apple sauce

    10 cherries mixed with handful of nuts (cashews, almonds, or walnuts)

    8 baby carrots with 2 tablespoons of hummus

Ants on a log (2 celery sticks dabbed with 1 tablespoon of raw nut butter and 1 tablespoon organic
raisins)

1 piece of medium-size fruit

Small beet salad

1 cup of beet juice

20 almonds

Small fruit cup

8 halves of dried apricots

2 tablespoons of sunflower seeds

4 slices of Melba whole-wheat or whole-grain toast

MEAL 2

- 1 cup of hibiscus tea (can be consumed either cold or
  hot)
- Choose one of the following:

  3 servings of vegetables (Remember, a serving is
  about the size of the average person's fist.)

  1 large green garden salad (no croutons, no bacon
  bits, 4 tablespoons of fat-free or low-fat dressing)

  1 protein shake (200 calories or less)

  1 bowl of soup (200 calories or less; no potatoes, no
  cream). Good choices are chicken noodle, vegetable, lentil, chickpea, split pea, black bean, tomato
  bisque, etc. Be careful of sodium content!

- If you choose the protein shake or soup, you should
  also consume 1 serving of veggies

- You can choose one of the following beverages in addition to the tea:

  One 12-ounce can of diet soda

  1 cup of lemonade (freshly squeezed preferred)

Unlimited plain water (flat or fizzy)

1 cup of flavored water

1 cup of juice (not from concentrate)

1 cup of unsweetened iced tea

1 cup of low-fat, reduced-fat, or fat-free milk, unsweetened soy milk, or unsweetened almond milk

SNACK 2

- Choose one of the following:

  Raw trail mix (½ cup of raw nuts with sunflower or pumpkin seeds and dried fruit)

  2 dates stuffed with almonds (take out the pit and replace with a few almonds)

  ½ cup raisins, raw walnuts, and pinch of sea salt (mix together)

  3 tomato slices and fresh basil drizzled with olive oil

  ½ cucumber, sliced, sprinkled with pinch of sea salt and fat-free vinaigrette dressing

  1 cup of unsweetened apple sauce

  10 cherries mixed with handful of nuts (cashews, almonds, or walnuts)

  8 baby carrots with 2 tablespoons of hummus

  Ants on a log (2 celery sticks dabbed with 1 tablespoon of raw nut butter and 1 tablespoon organic raisins)

  1 piece of medium-size fruit

  Small beet salad

  1 cup of beet juice

  20 almonds

  Small fruit cup

  8 halves of dried apricots

2 tablespoons of sunflower seeds

4 slices of Melba whole-wheat or whole-grain toast

MEAL 3

- 1 cup of 100-percent fresh cranberry juice (not from concentrate, no additives); mix with a little water to reduce the bitterness

- Choose one of the following:

    1 veggie burger (3½ inches in diameter, ½-inch thick)

    5-ounce piece of lean beef (no frying)

    5-ounce piece of chicken (no skin, no frying)

    5-ounce piece of fish (no frying)

    5-ounce piece of turkey (no skin, no frying)

    1 cup of spaghetti and meatballs

    (5 ounces is about the size of a deck and a half of playing cards.)

- 1 serving of veggies

- Half of a baked sweet potato (no whipped cream or other additions; you can add 1 teaspoon of butter) *or* ½ cup of cooked rice (brown preferred, but you can have white if you choose)

- You can choose one of the following beverages in addition to the cranberry juice:

    1 cup of lemonade (freshly squeezed preferred)

    Unlimited plain water (flat or fizzy)

    1 cup of flavored water

    1 cup of juice (not from concentrate)

    1 cup of unsweetened iced tea

    1 cup of low-fat, reduced-fat, or fat-free milk, unsweetened soy milk, or unsweetened almond milk

SNACK 3

- Choose one of the following:

  Raw trail mix (½ cup of raw nuts with sunflower or pumpkin seeds and dried fruit)

  2 dates stuffed with almonds (take out the pit and replace with a few almonds)

  ½ cup raisins, raw walnuts, and pinch of sea salt (mix together)

  3 tomato slices and fresh basil drizzled with olive oil

  ½ cucumber, sliced, sprinkled with pinch of sea salt and fat-free vinaigrette dressing

  1 cup of unsweetened apple sauce

  10 cherries mixed with handful of nuts (cashews, almonds, or walnuts)

  8 baby carrots with 2 tablespoons of hummus

  Ants on a log (2 celery sticks dabbed with 1 tablespoon of raw nut butter and 1 tablespoon organic raisins)

  1 piece of medium-size fruit

  Small beet salad

  1 cup of beet juice

  20 almonds

  Small fruit cup

  8 halves of dried apricots

  2 tablespoons of sunflower seeds

  4 slices of Melba whole-wheat or whole-grain toast

MEAL 4

- Choose one of the following. Your choice must be 200 calories or less and no sugar added.

    1 fruit smoothie

    1 protein shake

    1 veggie smoothie

- 1 cup of beans or other legumes (no baked beans)
- Choose one of the following beverages:

    1 cup of lemonade (freshly squeezed preferred)

    Unlimited plain water (flat or fizzy)

    1 cup of flavored water

    1 cup of juice (not from concentrate)

    1 cup of unsweetened iced tea

    1 cup of low-fat, reduced-fat, or fat-free milk, unsweetened soy milk, or unsweetened almond milk

EXERCISE

- Amount of exercise today: Minimum 30 minutes. If you want to do more, all the better! Work as hard as you can!
- Choose a combination of the items below to fulfill your exercise requirement:

    15 minutes jogging outside

    15 minutes walking/running on treadmill

    15 minutes on elliptical machine

    15 minutes on stationary or mobile bicycle

    15 minutes swimming laps

    15 minutes on stair climber

    225 jump rope revolutions

    20 minutes treadmill intervals

    15 minutes of Zumba

    15 minutes of spinning

    15 minutes of any other high-intensity cardio

    15 minutes of rowing machine

SHRED WEEK 6, DAY 6

MEAL 1

- 1 piece of fruit (choose a pear or apple or orange if possible)
- Choose one of the following:

    1 grilled cheese sandwich on 100-percent whole-grain or 100-percent whole-wheat bread

    1 small bowl of oatmeal (1 ½ cups cooked)

    2 egg whites *or* 1 egg-white omelet with diced veggies (made with 2 egg whites max)

    1 small bowl of sugar-free cereal with fat-free, skim, or 1-percent fat milk

    2 pancakes plus 2 strips of bacon (pancakes should be no larger than a CD; no more than 1½ tablespoons syrup, 1 pat of butter; try turkey bacon)

    1 small bowl of Cream of Wheat (1 cup cooked)

- 1 cup of fresh grapefruit, apple, or orange juice

SNACK 1

- 150 calories

MEAL 2

- 1 cup of hibiscus tea (can be consumed either cold or hot)
- Choose one of the following:

    3 servings of vegetables (Remember, a serving is about the size of the average person's fist.)

    1 large green garden salad (no croutons, no bacon

bits, 4 tablespoons of fat-free or low-fat dressing)

1 protein shake (200 calories or less)

1 bowl of soup (200 calories or less; no potatoes, no cream). Good choices are chicken noodle, vegetable, lentil, chickpea, split pea, black bean, tomato bisque, etc. Be careful of sodium content!

- If you choose the protein shake or soup, you should also consume 1 serving of veggies
- You can choose one of the following beverages in addition to the tea:

  One 12-ounce can of diet soda

  1 cup of lemonade (freshly squeezed preferred)

  Unlimited plain water (flat or fizzy)

  1 cup of flavored water

  1 cup of juice (not from concentrate)

  1 cup of unsweetened iced tea

  1 cup of low-fat, reduced-fat, or fat-free milk, unsweetened soy milk, or unsweetened almond milk

SNACK 2

- Choose one of the following:

  Raw trail mix (½ cup of raw nuts with sunflower or pumpkin seeds and dried fruit)

  2 dates stuffed with almonds (take out the pit and replace with a few almonds)

  ½ cup raisins, raw walnuts, and pinch of sea salt (mix together)

  3 tomato slices and fresh basil drizzled with olive oil

  ½ cucumber, sliced, sprinkled with pinch of sea salt and fat-free vinaigrette dressing

1 cup of unsweetened apple sauce

10 cherries mixed with handful of nuts (cashews, almonds, or walnuts)

8 baby carrots with 2 tablespoons of hummus

Ants on a log (2 celery sticks dabbed with 1 tablespoon of raw nut butter and 1 tablespoon organic raisins)

1 piece of medium-size fruit

Small beet salad

1 cup of beet juice

20 almonds

Small fruit cup

8 halves of dried apricots

2 tablespoons of sunflower seeds

4 slices of Melba whole-wheat or whole-grain toast

MEAL 3

- Choose one of the following:

    1 veggie burger (3½ inches in diameter, ½-inch thick)

    5-ounce piece of lean beef (no frying)

    5-ounce piece of chicken (no skin, no frying)

    5-ounce piece of fish (no frying)

    5-ounce piece of turkey (no skin, no frying)

    1 cup of spaghetti and meatballs

    (5 ounces is about the size of a deck and a half of playing cards.)

- 1 serving of veggies

- Half of a baked sweet potato (no whipped cream or other additions; you can add 1 teaspoon of butter) *or* ½ cup of cooked rice (brown preferred, but you can have white if you choose)

- Choose one of the following:

    1 cup of lemonade (freshly squeezed preferred)

    Unlimited plain water (flat or fizzy)

    1 cup of flavored water

    1 cup of juice (not from concentrate)

    1 cup of unsweetened iced tea

    1 cup of low-fat, reduced-fat, or fat-free milk, unsweetened soy milk, or unsweetened almond milk

SNACK 3

- 150 calories

MEAL 4

- 1 large green garden salad (no croutons, no bacon bits, 4 tablespoons of fat-free or low-fat dressing)
- 1 cup of soup
- Choose one of the following beverages. Choose a different beverage from what you chose in meal 3.

    1 cup of lemonade (freshly squeezed preferred)

    Unlimited plain water (flat or fizzy)

    1 cup of flavored water

    1 cup of juice (not from concentrate)

    1 cup of unsweetened iced tea

    1 cup of low-fat, reduced-fat, or fat-free milk, unsweetened soy milk, or unsweetened almond milk

EXERCISE

- Rest Day. But if you're inspired to do something, by all means go and do it. Every minute of exercise burns more calories and gets you closer to your goal. You might even try playing a sport, which can be a fun way to burn calories without feeling like you're actually working out.

SHRED WEEK 6, DAY 7

MEAL 1

- 1 cup of lemon water. Pour 8 ounces of water, either hot or cold. Squeeze the juice from half a lemon directly into the water. If you like, add ½ teaspoon of sugar. Mix well and drink.

- 1 piece of fruit. This can be 1 banana, 1 apple, 1 pear, etc. It can also be ½ cup of raspberries, blueberries, blackberries, or strawberries.

- Choose one of the following. Your portion should be 1 cup cooked.

    1 small bowl of oatmeal

    1 small bowl of Cream of Wheat

    1 small bowl of grits

- 1 cup of fresh juice *not* from concentrate (grapefruit, apple, orange juice, tomato, carrot, etc.)

SNACK 1

- 100 calories or less

MEAL 2

- Choose one of the following. Your choice must be 200 calories or less.

    1 fruit smoothie

    1 protein shake

    1 bowl of soup (no potatoes, no cream). Good choices are chicken noodle, vegetable, lentil, chickpea, split pea, black bean, tomato bisque, etc. Be careful of sodium content!

- 1 piece of fruit *or* 1 serving of veggies
- Choose one of the following beverages:

    One 12-ounce can of diet soda

    1 cup of lemonade (freshly squeezed preferred)

    Unlimited plain water (flat or fizzy)

    1 cup of flavored water

    1 cup of juice (not from concentrate)

    1 cup of unsweetened iced tea

SNACK 2

- 150 calories or less

MEAL 3

- Choose one of the following. Your choice must not exceed 200 calories. Try to choose something different from what you had in meal 2 if you can. You don't have to, but try.

    1 milk shake

    1 fruit smoothie

    1 protein shake

    1 veggie shake (You can use any veggies you want.)

    1 bowl of soup (no potatoes, no cream). Good choices are chicken noodle, vegetable, lentil, chickpea, split pea, black bean, tomato bisque, etc. Be careful of sodium content!

- Choose one from the following beverages. Choose a different beverage from what you chose with meal 2.

One 12-ounce can of diet soda

1 cup of lemonade (freshly squeezed preferred)

Unlimited plain water (flat or fizzy)

1 cup of flavored water

1 cup of juice (not from concentrate)

1 cup of unsweetened iced tea

SNACK 3

- 100 calories or less

MEAL 4

- Choose from Group A *or* Group B. *Do not* choose from both:

    Group A—choose one of the following:

    5-ounce piece of chicken (no skin, no frying)

    5-ounce piece of fish (no frying)

    5-ounce piece of turkey (no skin, no frying)

    All of the above come with ½ cup of cooked brown rice and 1 serving of veggies.

    Group B—you can have both items below:

    1 serving of lasagna (with or without meat), 4 inches × 2 inches × 1 inch

    1 serving of veggies

- Choose one of the following beverages. Choose something different from what you chose with meals 2 and 3.

    One 12-ounce can of diet soda

    1 cup of lemonade (freshly squeezed preferred)

    Unlimited plain water (flat or fizzy)

    1 cup of flavored water

    1 cup of juice (not from concentrate)

    1 cup of unsweetened iced tea

EXERCISE

- Amount of exercise today: Minimum 30 minutes. If you want to do more, all the better! Work as hard as you can!

- Choose a combination of the items below to fulfill your exercise requirement:

  15 minutes jogging outside

  15 minutes walking/running on treadmill

  15 minutes on elliptical machine

  15 minutes on stationary or mobile bicycle

  15 minutes swimming laps

  15 minutes on stair climber

  225 jump rope revolutions

  20 minutes treadmill intervals

  15 minutes of Zumba

  15 minutes of spinning

  15 minutes of any other high-intensity cardio

  15 minutes of rowing machine

CHAPTER 9

SHRED Snacks

This chapter is just as critical to the SHRED program as the others. Snacks figure heavily into the success of this plan. Many people don't understand snacks. The SHRED program sets the record straight and demonstrates how snacks can help you lose weight rather than gain it. The key to making the most out of snacks is understanding that snacks are not meals: they are bridges between meals. Many people consume an entire meal's worth of calories in a "snack," when in reality they've simply eaten another meal.

Successful weight loss involves many different factors, but one factor that remains paramount is calories. Making sure you don't overindulge in calories is critical to ultimate success. One area where many people make a mistake is with snacks. Consuming too many calories while snacking only increases your day's total calorie count, and this will inevitably lead to weight gain and program failure. Snacks are not mandatory on the SHRED plan, but they are heavily encouraged because they can prevent hunger pangs and prevent you from consuming too many calories at the next meal.

Snacks are also helpful because of a concept I like to call "calorie distribution." I will demonstrate this concept through an illustration. Take two people, Clara and Joan. They both consume 2,000 calories each day. However, they consume their calories differently. Clara consumes most of her calories in the first half of the day, but Joan consumes hers during the second half.

CLARA

8:00 A.M.–3:00 P.M.	3:00 P.M.–10:00 P.M.
1200 cals	800 cals

JOAN

8:00 A.M.–3:00 P.M.	3:00 P.M.–10:00 P.M.
800 cals	1200 cals

Clara also distributes her calories differently. She eats 4 meals, and 3 snacks. Joan eats only 3 meals and 2 snacks.

	Meal 1	Snack 1	Meal 2	Snack 2	Meal 3	Meal 4	Snack 3
Clara	450 cals	100 cals	450 cals	150 cals	400 cals	350 cals	100 cals

	Meal 1	Snack 1	Meal 2	Snack 2	Meal 3
Joan	300 cal	300 cal	500 cal	300 cal	600 cal

In the above example, while the women both eat the same total number of calories in any given day, research has shown that distributing the calories over more meals and snacks is advantageous in keeping hormone levels even. So it's not always how much you eat, but how you eat your foods that matters. Choose snacks from the items listed in this chapter or outside of the list as long as you stay within the calorie counts. Snacking is completely fine and should be enjoyed, but remember that it's only a bridge between meals, a means to quiet hunger pangs until you consume your next meal. Don't overindulge, but choose strategically, and snacking will help you reach your goals.

Following are two grab-bag lists of snacks at both 150 and 100 calories. Grab any of them to help satisfy the snack requirements in each week of the cycle.

150-CALORIE SNACKS

▶ 20 grapes with 15 peanuts
▶ 1 mozzarella cheese stick and 7 TLC Honey Sesame Crackers
▶ Applesauce and cereal: 1 applesauce pouch and ½ cup of dry cereal
▶ Hummus and cucumbers: cut up half of a large cucumber and combine it with 2 tablespoons of hummus
▶ Kiwi and oats: Slice a kiwi with a ½ cup of oat cereal
▶ Sliced banana with three Triscuits
▶ ¾ cup of steamed edamame (baby soybeans)
▶ Watermelon skewers: take 6 toothpicks and on each place 1 cube watermelon, 1 small cube feta cheese, and 1 slice cucumber

- Strawberries and chocolate: 1 cup whole strawberries dipped in 1 tablespoon melted semisweet chocolate chips
- 1 18 Rabbits Bunny Bar
- 45 shelled pistachios
- 1 medium apple with 1 tablespoon natural peanut butter
- 8 Kashi Wheat Thins with a light cheese wedge from Laughing Cow
- 1 cup snap peas with 3 tablespoons hummus
- 1 medium pear and 1 cup of low-fat or skim milk
- 3 rye crackers or Wheat Thins and 2 tablespoons spreadable "light" cheese
- Baby burrito: 6-inch corn tortilla, 2 tablespoons bean dip, and 2 tablespoons salsa
- Minestrone soup: ½ can of minestrone soup and 2 teaspoons grated parmesan cheese
- ¼ cup low-fat cottage cheese and ¼ cup fresh pineapple
- 1 packet Quaker's Low Sugar Instant Oatmeal (prepare with water)
- ½ cup roasted pumpkin seeds (keep in shells)
- 7 olives stuffed with 1 tablespoon blue cheese
- Brown rice vegetable sushi rolls, 5 pieces
- 1-ounce pretzels and 1 teaspoon French's Honey Mustard
- 2 squares of graham crackers and 8 ounces of skim milk
- 4 turkey slices and 1 medium apple, sliced
- ½ medium avocado sprinkled with sea salt
- Small baked potato topped with salsa

- ▶ 1 cup yogurt parfait and 1 tablespoon of granola
- ▶ 15 cashews, roasted and salted
- ▶ 1 Skinny Cow Ice Cream Sandwich
- ▶ 1 small container of tapioca pudding
- ▶ 1 medium papaya with a squeeze of lime juice on top
- ▶ 15 baked Tostitos Scoops and 2 tablespoons bean dip
- ▶ Peanut butter and jelly: ½ whole-grain English muffin, 1 tablespoon peanut butter, and sugar-free jelly
- ▶ 10 walnut halves and 1 sliced kiwi
- ▶ English muffin pizza: whole-wheat English muffin topped with 1 tablespoon of tomato sauce, 1 tablespoon low-fat cheese of your choice, and 1 tablespoon of parmesan cheese. Broil.
- ▶ Egg salad: 1 whole egg, ½ teaspoon low-fat mayo, and spices spread on half of a toasted whole-wheat or whole-grain bagel
- ▶ Cottage cheese and almond butter: ½ cup no-salt added 1-percent cottage cheese mixed with 1 tablespoon almond butter
- ▶ 5 pitted dates stuffed with 5 whole almonds
- ▶ Blueberries and sorbet: ½ cup fruit sorbet topped with ½ cup blueberries
- ▶ 10 baby carrots dipped in 2 tablespoons of lite salad dressing
- ▶ Turkey wrap: 2 slices of deli turkey breast, whole-grain flatbread, sliced tomatoes, cucumbers, and lettuce

- ▶ 1 Quaker breakfast bar
- ▶ 4 Nabisco ginger snap cookies
- ▶ 1 Nature Valley Oats 'n Honey crunchy granola bar
- ▶ ¾ cup halved strawberries topped with 3 tablespoons light Cool Whip
- ▶ 1 medium mango
- ▶ 6 dried figs
- ▶ Loaded pepper slices: 1 cup red bell pepper slices topped with ¼ cup warmed black beans and 1 tablespoon guacamole
- ▶ 1 small baked potato topped with a mixture of salsa and 1 tablespoon of low-fat cheddar cheese
- ▶ 1½ cups of diced watermelon
- ▶ 1 can of tuna, drained, season to taste
- ▶ 2 frozen fruit bars
- ▶ 4 pot stickers dipped in 2 teaspoons of reduced-sodium soy sauce
- ▶ ¾ cup of roasted cauliflower, pinch of sea salt
- ▶ 1 Mother Earth fruit crumble bar
- ▶ Roasted chickpeas: ½ cup of chickpeas tossed with 2 tablespoons of olive oil; spread on cookie sheet and lightly salted; bake at 350 degrees for 12–15 minutes
- ▶ 12 baked tortilla chips and ½ cup salsa
- ▶ 21 raw almonds
- ▶ Stuffed tomatoes: 10 halved grape tomatoes stuffed with a mixture of ¼ cup low-fat ricotta cheese, 1 tablespoon diced black olives, and a pinch of black pepper

- ▶ ½ cup of no-sugar-added applesauce mixed with 10 pecan halves
- ▶ 2 tablespoons hummus spread on 4 crackers
- ▶ 1 Kashi Honey Almond Flax Chewy Granola Bar
- ▶ 1½ strips low-fat string cheese
- ▶ 2 ounces of turkey jerky
- ▶ Slightly more than ¼ cup of dried apricots
- ▶ ½ cup shelled pistachios
- ▶ 2 scoops of sorbet
- ▶ 9 pieces of chocolate-covered almonds
- ▶ Frozen banana slices
- ▶ Chocolate-dipped pretzels: 3 honey pretzel sticks dipped in semisweet chocolate morsels melted in a microwave. Once covered in chocolate, put pretzels in freezer until chocolate sets.
- ▶ 1 small chocolate pudding
- ▶ 4 chocolate-chip cookies, each a little larger than the size of poker chips
- ▶ 50 Pepperidge Farm Goldfish
- ▶ 9 Ritz crackers
- ▶ 12 saltines
- ▶ 4 saltine jelly sandwiches: take 8 saltines, spread sugar-free jelly on half of them, and cover with the other halves
- ▶ 5 Ritz crackers slightly smeared with peanut butter
- ▶ 1 cup of grape tomatoes
- ▶ ½ blueberry muffin
- ▶ 1 Jell-O Chocolate Fudge Sugar-Free Pudding with 5 sliced strawberries and 1 tablespoon of whipped cream

- ▶ 2 cups of air-popped popcorn sprinkled with parmesan cheese
- ▶ 1½ cups of frozen grapes
- ▶ Mediterranean salad: dice 1 tomato, 1 medium cucumber, ½ red onion. Sprinkle with 2 tablespoons low-fat feta cheese.
- ▶ Watermelon treat: 1 cup of diced watermelon topped with 2 tablespoons of crumbled feta cheese
- ▶ 1 large apple, sliced, sprinkled with cinnamon
- ▶ Tasty pepper: slice bell pepper, marinate in 1 tablespoon of balsamic vinegar, salt, and pepper
- ▶ 2 Vlasic Kosher Dill pickle spears
- ▶ Tuna salad: 1 can of light tuna in water, mix in 1 tablespoon low-fat mayo, and 1 diced sweet pickle
- ▶ 1 cup of Cheerios
- ▶ 2 Dole fruit juice bars
- ▶ 1 Nestle Crunch reduced-fat ice-cream bar
- ▶ ½ cup Breyers Light Natural Vanilla ice cream
- ▶ 1 Quaker Chewy Peanut Butter & Chocolate Chunk granola bar
- ▶ 1 Nature Valley Crunchy Peanut Butter granola bar
- ▶ ⅛ loaf of Entenmann's Light Golden Loaf cake
- ▶ ⅛ loaf of Entenmann's Light Chocolate Loaf cake
- ▶ 2 Popsicles
- ▶ 2 Fudgsicles

100-CALORIE SNACKS

▶ Chocolate banana: ½ frozen banana dipped in two squares of melted dark chocolate

▶ ½ cup nonfat Greek yogurt with dash cinnamon and 1 teaspoon honey

▶ 2 ¼-inch-thick pineapple rounds, grilled or sautéed

▶ 1 cup blueberries with 2 tablespoons whipped topping

▶ Stuffed figs: 2 small dried figs stuffed with 1 tablespoon reduced-fat ricotta and sprinkled with cinnamon

▶ Citrus-berry salad: 1 cup mixed berry salad (raspberries, strawberries, blueberries, and blackberries) tossed with 1 tablespoon fresh-squeezed orange juice

▶ 2 graham cracker squares and 1 teaspoon peanut butter, sprinkled with cinnamon

▶ 10 baby carrots with 2 tablespoons hummus

▶ Cheesy breaded tomatoes: 2 roasted plum tomatoes sliced and topped with 2 tablespoons bread crumbs and a sprinkle of parmesan cheese

▶ Kale chips: ½ cup raw kale (stems removed) baked with 1 teaspoon olive oil at 400 degrees until crisp

▶ Cucumber sandwich: ½ English muffin with 2 tablespoons cottage cheese and 3 slices cucumber

▶ ⅓ cup wasabi peas

▶ Cucumber salad: 1 large cucumber (sliced) with 2 tablespoons red onion and 2 tablespoons apple cider vinegar

▶ Chickpea salad: ¼ cup chickpeas with 1 tablespoon

sliced scallions, a squeeze of lemon juice, and ¼ cup diced tomatoes

▶ 15 mini pretzel sticks with 2 tablespoons fat-free cream cheese

▶ Spicy black beans: ¼ cup black beans with 1 tablespoon salsa and 1 tablespoon nonfat Greek yogurt

▶ About 40 Pepperidge Farm Goldfish

▶ 1 nonfat mozzarella cheese stick with half of a baseball-size apple, sliced

▶ 3 dried apricots stuffed with 1 tablespoon crumbled blue cheese

▶ Tropical cottage cheese: ½ cup nonfat cottage cheese with ½ cup fresh mango and pineapple, chopped

▶ Strawberry salad: 1 cup raw spinach with ½ cup sliced strawberries and 1 tablespoon balsamic vinegar

▶ Crunchy kale salad: 1 cup kale leaves chopped with 1 teaspoon honey and 1 tablespoon balsamic vinegar

▶ Turkey roll-ups: 4 slices smoked turkey rolled up and dipped in 2 teaspoons honey mustard

▶ Greek tomatoes: 1 tomato (about the size of a tennis ball) chopped and mixed with 1 tablespoon feta and a squeeze of lemon juice

▶ ¼ cup low-fat granola

▶ ½ cup oat cereal, toasted

▶ 1 ½ cups puffed rice

▶ ½ cup Raisin Bran

▶ 7 animal crackers, plain

▶ 1½ sheets graham crackers

▶ ½ sheet matzoh

- ▶ 25 oyster crackers
- ▶ 7 saltines
- ▶ ¾ cup carrots, cooked
- ▶ 1 large carrot, raw
- ▶ 2 stalks celery, raw
- ▶ 1 medium cucumber, raw
- ▶ 1 cup lettuce, raw, drizzled with 2 tablespoons fat-free dressing
- ▶ 1 potato, baked (2 ounces)
- ▶ ½ cup potatoes, mashed with milk and butter
- ▶ 1 medium tomato, raw, pinch of salt
- ▶ 6 large clams
- ▶ 3 ounces cod, cooked
- ▶ 3 ounces crab, fresh, cooked
- ▶ ½ cup crab, canned
- ▶ 1 ½ ounces halibut, Atlantic fresh, cooked
- ▶ 2 ounces lobster, cooked
- ▶ 2 ounces mussels, cooked
- ▶ 6 oysters
- ▶ 2 ounces salmon, Atlantic fresh, cooked
- ▶ 2 ounces salmon, smoked
- ▶ 2 ounces scallops, bay, cooked
- ▶ 4 large scallops, sea, cooked
- ▶ 2 ounces tuna, yellowfin fresh, cooked
- ▶ 3 ounces tuna, canned in water
- ▶ 14 almonds
- ▶ 10 cashews
- ▶ 2 tablespoons flaxseeds
- ▶ 25 peanuts, dry-roasted
- ▶ 24 peanuts, oil-roasted

- 17 pecans
- 2 tablespoons poppy seeds
- 2 tablespoons pumpkin seeds
- 2 tablespoons sunflower seeds
- 6 dried apricots
- Sugar-free Jell-O with one scoop ice cream
- 25 cherries
- 1 Special K Chocolate Chip Cereal Bar
- 1 cup tomato bisque soup
- 3 crackers lightly spread with peanut butter
- 3 medium breadsticks with hummus
- 1 hard-boiled egg, salt and pepper to taste
- 2 small peaches
- 1 cup of strawberries
- 1 small baked potato
- 1 medium corn on the cob with seasoning
- 30 grapes
- ½ cup of unsweetened applesauce with 1 slice of whole-wheat toast, cut into 4 strips for dunking
- 4–6 ounces of nonfat or low-fat yogurt
- 3 pineapple rings in natural juices
- 3 oven-baked potato wedges
- 1 rice cake with 1 tablespoon guacamole
- 1 cup of radishes, sliced or chopped
- 4 slices of Oscar Mayer fat-free bologna
- fat- and sugar-free frozen yogurt
- Artichokes, 16 calories each
- 1 cup of sliced zucchini, season to taste
- 1 cup of chicken noodle soup
- ½ cup clam chowder

- ▶ ¾ cup minestrone soup
- ▶ 1 nectarine
- ▶ 1½ cups sugar snap peas
- ▶ 2 slices of deli turkey breast
- ▶ 1 medium tomato sliced with a sprinkle of feta cheese and olive oil
- ▶ 8 small shrimps and 3 tablespoons cocktail sauce
- ▶ 1 tablespoon peanuts and 2 tablespoons dried cranberries
- ▶ 1 cup raspberries with 2 tablespoons plain yogurt
- ▶ 20 olives
- ▶ 1 cup miso soup
- ▶ 3 celery sticks stuffed with cottage cheese
- ▶ Portobello mushroom stuffed with roasted veggies and 1 teaspoon shredded low-fat cheese
- ▶ Medium grapefruit sprinkled with ½ teaspoon sugar
- ▶ 6 figs
- ▶ 20 grapes with 15 peanuts
- ▶ ½ pound fruit salad
- ▶ 4 dates
- ▶ 1 small baked sweet potato
- ▶ 1 can low-sodium V-8 100% Vegetable Juice
- ▶ 1 fresh pomegranate
- ▶ 3 cups of air-popped popcorn
- ▶ 2 cups broccoli florets
- ▶ 1 large cucumber, sliced
- ▶ 1 strip of low-fat string cheese
- ▶ Black bean salsa over 3 eggplant slices
- ▶ 2 ounces of lean roast beef
- ▶ 1 seven-grain Belgian waffle

▸ 4 mini rice cakes with 2 tablespoons low-fat cottage cheese
▸ 1 Nabisco 100 Calorie Packs Mister Salty Milk Chocolate–Covered Pretzels
▸ 1 Kraft Handi-Snacks Chocolate Pudding

CHAPTER 10

SHRED Smoothie Recipes

Smoothies are spectacular. They are a convenient and tasty way to eat fruits and vegetables and their calorie counts can be tightly controlled. Throughout the SHRED program you are given options to choose a smoothie for certain meals. Making your own smoothie is quite simple with an inexpensive blender. Most of these recipes take no more than five minutes from start to finish. You might not always be able to make your own smoothie. It's completely fine, of course, to get them made for you, but make sure the calorie count fits with what is recommended in the menu. Keep track of this, it is important.

When you make your own smoothie, make sure you pay attention to how many servings the recipe makes. Some will make two servings or more, while some will make one. You are only supposed to consume one serving for a meal. So if the recipe makes more than one, put the rest in a storage container and refrigerate it for later.

Follow the recipes as closely as possible. You might be tempted to add sugar, but try not to. If you must, don't add more than a teaspoon in recipes that make two servings or more. Some recipes might call for sugar. It's fine to use it in those recipes. Most important, experiment by switching the fruits and combining flavors. There is a lot of taste flexibility when it comes to blending your own smoothie.

NOTE: For all recipes that call for milk, you can use skim, reduced, soy, almond, or goat's milk.

Frozen fruit can be used as long as it contains no added sugars.

• STRAWBERRY PEACH SMOOTHIE •

TOTAL TIME: 10 MINUTES

SERVINGS: 1

UNDER 200 CALORIES

¼ cup vanilla-flavored soy milk or low-fat milk

1 scoop (½ cup) low-fat vanilla ice cream

½ cup frozen sliced strawberries or ½ cup fresh sliced strawberries and 4 ice cubes

1 small fresh peach, peeled and sliced

Pour milk into a blender and add ice cream, frozen strawberries or fresh strawberries and ice, and peach slices. Blend until smooth and creamy.

• FRUIT POWER SMOOTHIE •

TOTAL TIME: 5 MINUTES

SERVINGS: 4

UNDER 200 CALORIES

1 cup strawberries

½ cup blueberries

1 kiwi, peeled and sliced

1 banana, peeled and
  chopped

1 cup ice cubes

One 8-ounce container
  peach yogurt

½ cup orange juice, not from
  concentrate

In a blender, blend the strawberries, blueberries, kiwi, banana, ice, yogurt, and orange juice until smooth.

• TASTY AND HEALTHY SMOOTHIE •

TOTAL TIME: 10 MINUTES

SERVINGS: 1

UNDER 200 CALORIES

½ frozen banana, peeled
   and chopped
½ cup frozen strawberries
1½ tablespoons flaxseed

½ cup fat-free plain yogurt
½ cup nonfat milk
1 teaspoon honey

Place all ingredients in a blender and purée until smooth.

• STRAWBERRY-PINEAPPLE SMOOTHIE •

TOTAL TIME: 5 MINUTES

SERVINGS: 2

UNDER 200 CALORIES

1 cup frozen strawberries

¾ cup pineapple juice, not
   from concentrate

¾ cup milk

1 tablespoon white sugar

½ cup vanilla yogurt

6 ice cubes

Blend the strawberries, pineapple juice, milk, sugar, vanilla yogurt, and ice in a blender until smooth.

• LEMON-BERRY SMOOTHIE •

TOTAL TIME: 5 MINUTES

SERVINGS: 4

UNDER 200 CALORIES

1 cup fresh blueberries

1 cup fresh strawberries

One 8-ounce container
   nonfat blueberry yogurt

1 ½ cups skim milk

1 cup ice cubes

Juice from ½ lemon

Place blueberries, strawberries, yogurt, milk, and ice cubes in a blender. Squeeze lemon juice into blender. Purée until smooth and creamy.

• BERRY DELICIOUS •

TOTAL TIME: 5 MINUTES

SERVINGS: 4

UNDER 200 CALORIES

2 cups frozen mixed berries
1 medium banana, peeled
   and sliced
1 cup milk

1 cup strawberry-flavored
   yogurt
½ teaspoon white sugar
   (optional)

Combine in a blender the mixed berries, banana, milk, strawberry yogurt, and sugar. Cover, and blend until smooth.

• SWEET BLACKBERRY SMOOTHIE •

TOTAL TIME: 5 MINUTES

SERVINGS: 1

UNDER 200 CALORIES

½ cup ice cubes
½ banana, peeled and
   sliced
½ cup yogurt

½ cup blackberries (fresh or
   frozen)
1 tablespoon of sugar
   (optional)

Blend the ice with the banana and yogurt until smooth. Add the blackberries and sugar and blend on low speed until smooth.

• JAZZY RAZZY RASPBERRY SMOOTHIE •

TOTAL TIME: 5 MINUTES

SERVINGS: 3

UNDER 200 CALORIES

1 cup fresh or frozen
   unsweetened raspberries
1 small ripe banana, peeled
   and cut into chunks

½ cup apple juice, not from
   concentrate
1 cup milk
½ cup raspberry yogurt

Combine all ingredients in a blender and purée until smooth.

• NO HASSLE MANGO SMOOTHIE •

TOTAL TIME: 5 MINUTES

SERVINGS: 1

UNDER 200 CALORIES

½ cup diced mangoes, frozen

3 tablespoons low-fat plain yogurt

⅔ cup skim milk

½ teaspoon sugar or ½ teaspoon honey

4 ice cubes

In a blender, combine frozen mango, yogurt, milk, and sugar or honey, with the ice cubes. Purée until mixture is smooth.

• CLASSIC BLUEBERRY-MANGO SMOOTHIE •

TOTAL TIME: 5 MINUTES

SERVINGS: 2

UNDER 200 CALORIES

1 cup frozen or fresh
blueberries

1 cup mango chunks

¼ cup vanilla soy milk,

almond milk, skim milk, or
water

1 cup plain yogurt

¼ cup ice chips, optional

Combine all ingredients in a blender, and purée until smooth.
If you use fresh blueberries the smoothie might be room temperature. Refrigerate until drink is desired temperature. If
you want to drink immediately, simply add ¼ cup ice chips
to the ingredients.

• ZIPPY APPLE-BERRY SMOOTHIE •

TOTAL TIME: 5 MINUTES

SERVINGS: 2

UNDER 200 CALORIES

½ cup strawberries, chopped (frozen optional)

½ cup blueberries

¼ cup plain low-fat yogurt

¾ cup apple juice, not from concentrate

2 cups ice chips

Combine all ingredients in a blender and purée on low speed until smooth.

• APPLE-BERRY EXTRAVAGANZA SMOOTHIE

•

TOTAL TIME: 5 MINUTES

SERVINGS: 4

UNDER 200 CALORIES

1 cup blueberries

1½ cups raspberries

2 apples, peeled, cored, and chopped

3 tablespoons white sugar, optional

1½ cups ice

½ cup low-fat vanilla yogurt

Combine all ingredients in a blender and purée until smooth.

• ORANGE-BERRY TWIST SMOOTHIE •

TOTAL TIME: 5 MINUTES

SERVINGS: 2

UNDER 200 CALORIES

2 navel oranges, peeled and seeds removed, cut into chunks

1 cup fresh or frozen raspberries

1 cup fresh or frozen blueberries

½ cup plain yogurt

½ cup of ice

Combine all ingredients in a blender and purée until smooth.

• SWEET DETOX SMOOTHIE •

TOTAL TIME: 5 MINUTES

SERVINGS: 2

UNDER 200 CALORIES

2 cups mixed frozen berries

1 pear, peeled, cored, and
    sliced

1 cup unsweetened pome-
    granate juice

1 cup ice

Combine all ingredients in a blender and purée until smooth.

• GREEN POWER MACHINE •

TOTAL TIME: 5 MINUTES

SERVINGS: 2

UNDER 200 CALORIES

½ cup apple, peeled, cored, and chopped

4 kale leaves, chopped

½ cup chopped mango

6 romaine leaves, chopped

¼ cup fresh parsley sprigs

1 inch fresh gingerroot, peeled and chopped

1 cup of water

Combine all ingredients in a blender and purée on low speed until smooth. Place in refrigerator. Serve chilled.

• OLD-FASHIONED STRAWBERRY-BANANA SMOOTHIE •

TOTAL TIME: 5 MINUTES

SERVINGS: 4

UNDER 200 CALORIES

3½ cups chopped strawber-
ries

3 bananas, peeled and
sliced

1½ cups plain low-fat yogurt

¼ cup orange juice, not from
concentrate

¼ cup milk or soy milk

1½ tablespoons honey

1 cup ice

Combine all ingredients in a blender and purée until smooth.

• THE DOWN UNDER •

TOTAL TIME: 5 MINUTES

SERVINGS: 2

UNDER 200 CALORIES

1 kiwi, peeled and chopped

½ cup chopped pineapple

1 orange, peeled, seeded, and chopped

1 small banana, peeled and sliced

7 strawberries, chopped

½ cup plain yogurt

1 cup of ice

Combine all ingredients in a blender and purée until smooth.

• THE OLD RELIABLE •

Apple-Banana Smoothie

TOTAL TIME: 5 MINUTES

SERVINGS: 2

UNDER 200 CALORIES

1 apple, peeled, cored, and chopped

1 banana, peeled and chopped

2 tablespoons plain low-fat yogurt

¼ cup milk

½ cup orange juice, not from concentrate

Combine all ingredients in a blender and purée on low speed until smooth.

• BANANA SHAKE •

TOTAL TIME: 5 MINUTES

SERVINGS: 1

250-300 CALORIES

1 whole banana, peeled and
   sliced
1 cup milk

¼ cup plain low-fat yogurt
¼ cup ice chips

Combine all ingredients in a blender and blend on medium
speed, creating a purée that's smooth and creamy.

• PURPLE POWER GRAPE SMOOTHIE •

TOTAL TIME: 5 MINUTES

SERVINGS: 2

UNDER 200 CALORIES

2 cups seedless black
   grapes
1 cup low-fat yogurt
1 cup milk

3 tablespoons sugar
½ cup ice cubes or crushed
   ice

Combine all ingredients in a blender. Blend on medium speed
until smooth and creamy.

• THE ENERGIZER BLUEBERRY-PEAR SMOOTHIE •

TOTAL TIME: 5 MINUTES

SERVINGS: 2

UNDER 200 CALORIES

1½ whole red pears
1 cup frozen blueberries
1 cup plain low-fat yogurt

1 teaspoon sugar
6 ice cubes

Cut the pears into chunks and remove the seeds and stems. Keep the skin on as it's full of healthy and tasty nutrients. Place all ingredients in a blender and purée on medium speed until smooth.

• FLUORESCENT PINEAPPLE-ORANGE SMOOTHIE •

TOTAL TIME: 5 MINUTES

SERVINGS: 1

250–300 CALORIES

1 cup pineapple chunks
½ frozen peeled banana,
    sliced

1 cup orange-tangerine juice
    blend, chilled
¼ cup carrot juice, chilled

Combine all ingredients in a blender and purée until smooth.

• THE VIRTUOSO •

Apple-Pear Smoothie

TOTAL TIME: 5 MINUTES

SERVINGS: 2

UNDER 200 CALORIES

1½ whole red apples

1 cup pear slices

1 cup plain low-fat yogurt

1 teaspoon sugar, optional

6 ice cubes

Core and cut apples into chunks. Keep the skin on as it's full of healthy and tasty nutrients. Place all ingredients in a blender and purée until smooth.

• LIGHT CUCUMBER SMOOTHIE •

TOTAL TIME: 7 MINUTES

SERVINGS: 2

UNDER 200 CALORIES

1 large garden cucumber,
  peeled, seeded, and cut
  into chunks (about
  1 cup)
½ cup frozen blueberries

½ cup plain or vanilla low-fat
  yogurt
½ tablespoon lemon juice
½ tablespoon lime juice
1 tablespoon honey

Combine all ingredients in a blender and purée until smooth.

• RASPBERRY-ORANGE ELIXIR •

TOTAL TIME: 7 MINUTES

SERVINGS: 2

UNDER 200 CALORIES

1 cup diced orange slices
1 cup raspberries
½ cup vanilla yogurt

1 tablespoon of sugar or
   honey
1 cup of ice

Combine all ingredients in a blender and purée until smooth.

• STRAWBERRY-PEACH-MANGO SMOOTHIE •

TOTAL TIME: 5 MINUTES

SERVINGS: 2

UNDER 200 CALORIES

1 cup frozen strawberries

1 peach, peeled, pitted, and sliced

1 cup mango chunks

¼ cup milk

1 cup plain yogurt

¼ cup ice chips, optional

Combine all ingredients in a blender and purée until smooth.

• THE TRIFECTA •

Strawberry-Peach-Carrot Smoothie

TOTAL TIME: 7 MINUTES

SERVINGS: 4

UNDER 200 CALORIES

1 cup frozen strawberries

1 medium carrot, peeled and sliced

1 peach, peeled, pitted, and sliced

½ cup plain or vanilla low-fat yogurt

½ tablespoon flaxseed oil

6 ice cubes

Combine all ingredients in a blender and purée until smooth.

• INVIGORATING APPLE-PEACH SMOOTHIE •

TOTAL TIME: 7 MINUTES

SERVINGS: 2

UNDER 200 CALORIES

1½ cups green apples, chopped

3 medium peaches, peeled, pitted, and sliced

1 teaspoon lime juice

½ cup plain low-fat yogurt

1 cup of ice

Combine all ingredients in a blender and purée until smooth.

• SWEET-AND-SOUR APPLE-CRANBERRY
SMOOTHIE •

TOTAL TIME: 7 MINUTES

SERVINGS: 2

250–300 CALORIES

1 ½ cups cranberries

1 large apple, peeled and
chopped

1 ½ cups plain low-fat yogurt

1 cup crushed ice

Combine all ingredients in a blender and purée until smooth.

• THE GRAZZY •
Grape-Raspberry Smoothie

TOTAL TIME: 5 MINUTES

SERVINGS: 2

UNDER 200 CALORIES

1 cup dark seedless grapes

1 cup frozen raspberries

½ cup plain low-fat yogurt

1 teaspoon sugar, optional

6 ice cubes

Combine all ingredients in a blender and purée until smooth.

CHAPTER 11

SHRED Protein Shake Recipes

• SUPER PROTEIN BLAST SHAKE •

TOTAL TIME: 5 MINUTES

SERVINGS: 2

200–250 CALORIES

¼ cup of vanilla whey protein powder (use whey isolate or hydrolyzed whey)

12 ounces almond milk (reduced-fat or fat-free cow's milk may be substituted)

4 frozen (or fresh) strawberries

¼ cup frozen (or fresh) blueberries

1 teaspoon honey

2 tablespoons low-fat vanilla yogurt

4 ice cubes

Add all ingredients to a blender. Blend on medium speed at first, then high speed until smooth and creamy.

• BLUE MANIA PROTEIN SHAKE •

TOTAL TIME: 5 MINUTES

SERVINGS: 2

200–250 CALORIES

¼ cup of vanilla whey protein powder (use whey isolate or hydrolyzed whey)

12 ounces almond milk (reduced-fat or fat-free cow's milk may be substituted)

¼ cup frozen (or fresh) blackberries

¾ cup frozen (or fresh) blueberries

2 tablespoons low-fat vanilla yogurt

½ teaspoon honey

4 ice cubes

Add all ingredients to a blender. Blend on medium speed at first, then high speed until smooth and creamy.

• CHOCOLATE LOVER'S PROTEIN SHAKE •

TOTAL TIME: 5 MINUTES

SERVINGS: 1

UNDER 200 CALORIES

¼ cup chocolate whey protein powder (use whey isolate or hydro-lyzed whey)

1 teaspoon powdered cocoa

½ medium peeled frozen banana, sliced

¼ cup low-fat or skim chocolate milk

¼ cup low-fat milk

4 ice cubes

Add all ingredients to a blender. Blend on medium speed at first, then high speed until smooth and creamy.

• RED REVOLUTION PROTEIN SHAKE •

TOTAL TIME: 5 MINUTES

SERVINGS: 2

200–250 CALORIES

¼ cup of vanilla whey protein powder (use whey isolate or hydrolyzed whey)

12 ounces almond milk (reduced-fat or fat-free cow's milk may be substituted)

4 frozen (or fresh) strawberries

½ cup frozen (or fresh) raspberries

1 teaspoon sugar (½ teaspoon agave nectar may be substituted)

2 tablespoons low-fat vanilla yogurt

4 ice cubes

Add all ingredients to a blender. Blend on medium speed at first, then high speed until smooth and creamy.

• TROPICAL SPLASH PROTEIN SHAKE •

TOTAL TIME: 5 MINUTES

SERVINGS: 2

200 CALORIES

¼ cup vanilla whey protein
   powder (use whey isolate
   or hydrolyzed whey)
1 cup frozen pineapple
½ cup frozen blueberries

¾ cup unsweetened vanilla
   almond milk
1 tablespoon unsweetened
   coconut milk

Add all ingredients to a blender. Blend on low to medium speed until smooth and creamy.

CHAPTER 12

SHRED Soup and Stew Recipes

Most of these simple, inexpensive recipes can be made in 30 minutes or less. You can use these recipes as a foundation and experiment by substituting ingredients. Just make sure you're staying mindful of the calories. For example, don't substitute a cream sauce for chicken broth. Soups and simple stews are a great way to fill up on fewer calories. If there are certain ingredients that you really don't like or are allergic to, feel free to customize the recipe within reason to fit your needs.

In these recipes your finished product will contain multiple servings. It is critical to remember that you are only to eat one serving at a particular meal. Whatever is left over, please place in a storage container and refrigerate it for later use. The serving for these soups and stews is between 1 and 1½ cups. If you consume within this range you'll be fine. *Bon appétit!*

• TRISTÉ'S CHICKEN NOODLE SOUP •

TOTAL TIME: 30 MINUTES

SERVINGS: 4

UNDER 200 CALORIES

1 ½ cups wide egg noodles

1 tablespoon butter

½ cup chopped onion

½ cup chopped celery

¾ cup sliced carrots

1 ½ cups diced, cooked chicken meat

6 cups chicken broth

1 ½ cups vegetable broth

¼ cup water

½ teaspoon dried basil

½ teaspoon dried oregano

1 teaspoon poultry seasoning

1 teaspoon salt

Salt and pepper to taste

Bring large pot of water to a boil. Add egg noodles and boil until tender, 5 to 10 minutes. Drain and set aside.

In a large pot, melt butter. Cook onion and celery in butter until tender. Don't overcook. Add carrots, chicken, chicken broth, vegetable broth, water, basil, oregano, poultry seasoning, salt, and pepper. Bring to a boil, then reduce heat and let simmer for 15 minutes before serving.

• BONNIE'S VEGETABLE SOUP •

TOTAL TIME: 30 MINUTES

SERVINGS: 4

UNDER 200 CALORIES

3 teaspoons olive oil

1 medium onion, diced

Kosher salt to taste

Pepper to taste

1 celery stalk, diced

2 medium carrots, diced

2 medium garlic cloves, peeled and minced

2 tablespoons flour

¼ cup corn kernels

¼ cup packed, chopped fresh parsley leaves

1 bay leaf (optional)

1 pinch dried thyme (optional)

3 cups chicken or vegetable broth

¾ pounds white potatoes, diced

¼ cup peas

¼ cup mushrooms

¼ cup red peppers chopped

1 cup peeled, seeded, and chopped tomatoes

Heat the olive oil in a large saucepan. Add the onion, season with salt and pepper. Stir in the celery, carrot, and garlic. Cook and stir until the veggies are tender and starting to brown, approximately 7 minutes. Add flour and cook another minute while stirring constantly. Season with salt and pepper.

Add the corn, parsley, bay leaf, and thyme, if using. Season again with salt and pepper and cook an additional 5 minutes.

Add the broth, potatoes, peas, mushrooms, peppers, and tomatoes. Bring the soup to a boil, then reduce the heat to low, allowing it to simmer, uncovered. Cook until the potatoes can be easily pierced with a fork, about 15 minutes. Remove bay leaf if using. Season with additional salt and pepper as needed and serve.

• BEAN, RICE, AND CHICKEN STEW •

TOTAL TIME: 60 MINUTES

SERVINGS: 2

200–300 CALORIES

4 ounces boneless, skinless chicken breast

2 cups cooked brown rice

½ cup cooked black or red beans or ½ cup canned black or red beans, rinsed and drained

½ cup chopped white onion

2 teaspoons ketchup

1 teaspoon Dijon mustard

1 teaspoon Worcestershire sauce

½ teaspoon brown sugar

Preheat the oven to 375°F.

Combine all ingredients in an oven-safe casserole dish and mix until well combined. Bake uncovered for 55 to 60 minutes and serve.

• WINTER CORN CHOWDER •

TOTAL TIME: 30 MINUTES

SERVINGS: 4

250–300 CALORIES

½ cup diced bacon

2 medium potatoes, peeled
   and chopped

½ medium onion, chopped

1½ cups cream-style corn

1 cup niblet corn

1 cup water

1 teaspoon salt

Ground black pepper to taste

1 cup whole milk

Cook bacon in a large pot until crisp. Drain and crumble bacon. Reserve about 1 tablespoon of drippings in the pot.

Add the potatoes and onion to the pot with the crumbled bacon and reserved drippings. Cook and stir for 5 minutes. Add the corn and water and season with salt and pepper. Bring soup to a boil, reduce heat, and let simmer for 15 minutes, covered. Keep stirring until potatoes are tender.

Warm the milk in a small saucepan. Add milk to the soup 5 minutes before it's done simmering. Serve.

• STURDY BLACK BEAN SOUP •

READY TIME: 30 MINUTES

SERVINGS: 4

250–300 CALORIES

2 tablespoons olive oil

1 medium onion, chopped

4 garlic cloves, peeled and
   minced

1 tablespoon cumin

One 15-ounce can black
   beans

3 tomatoes, chopped

3½ cups chicken broth

1 tablespoon lime juice (from
   one whole lime)

1 teaspoon ground black
   pepper

1 tablespoon minced fresh
   cilantro leaves

Heat olive oil in a large saucepan. Sauté onion, garlic, and
cumin for 3 to 5 minutes. Add beans, tomatoes, broth, lime
juice, and pepper. Bring to a boil, cover, reduce heat, and let
simmer for 7 minutes. Add cilantro. Serve.

• BIG BELL'S SWEET POTATO CARROT SOUP •

TOTAL TIME: 30 MINUTES

SERVINGS: 4

UNDER 200 CALORIES

1 tablespoon olive oil or butter

1 medium onion, chopped

1 clove garlic, peeled and minced

½ teaspoon salt

2 medium sweet potatoes, peeled and chopped

4 medium carrots, peeled and chopped

1 tablespoon ginger

1 cup low-sodium chicken or vegetable stock

2 cups water

¼ cup sour cream

In a large pot, heat oil or melt butter. Add onion, garlic, and salt. Cook until the onions are soft, about 3 minutes.

Add sweet potato, carrot, and ginger. Add stock and water. Bring to a boil. Reduce heat and simmer until all vegetables are very soft, about 15 minutes.

Strain vegetables and carefully put them in a blender. Purée until smooth. Add sour cream and blend. Taste and add more salt as needed. Serve.

• UNCLE JOHNNY'S WHITE BEAN SOUP •

TOTAL TIME: 30 MINUTES OR LESS

SERVINGS: 4

UNDER 200 CALORIES

2 cups of cannellini beans

1 strip of bacon, optional

4 tablespoons olive oil

1 medium onion, finely chopped

1½ celery stalks, finely chopped

½ carrot, finely chopped

One 15-ounce can plum tomatoes or stewed tomatoes

One 15-ounce can chicken or vegetable broth

Salt and pepper to taste

Purée one cup of beans in a food processor or blender.

Cook 1 strip of bacon and crumble, if using.

Heat oil in a large saucepan and add the onion, and cook until soft about 3 minutes. Add the celery, carrots, and tomatoes, and cook for 7 minutes more.

Warm the broth and pour it into the saucepan. Gradually stir in the beans and bean purée. Add the bacon. Let simmer for approximately 15 minutes. Season with salt and pepper. Serve.

• HEARTY SQUASH SOUP •

TOTAL TIME: 60 MINUTES

SERVINGS: 4

300 CALORIES

2 tablespoons butter

1 small onion, chopped

1 stalk celery, chopped

1 medium carrot, chopped

2 medium potatoes, cubed

1 medium butternut squash,

peeled, seeded, and
cubed

One 32-ounce container
chicken stock

Salt and freshly ground black
pepper to taste

Melt the butter in a large pot. Add the onion, celery, carrot, potatoes, and squash and cook for 5 minutes, or until onions are lightly browned. Pour in enough of the chicken stock to cover the vegetables. Bring to a boil. Reduce heat to low, cover pot, and simmer for 40 minutes, or until all vegetables are tender.

Carefully transfer the soup to a blender, and blend until smooth. Return the soup to the pot, and mix in any remaining stock to attain desired consistency. Season with salt and pepper and serve.

• LUSCIOUS TOMATO BISQUE SOUP •

TOTAL TIME: 30 MINUTES

SERVINGS: 4

UNDER 200 CALORIES

2 garlic cloves, peeled and minced

4 tablespoons butter

3 tablespoons all-purpose flour

3 cups chicken broth

9 ounces tomato paste

1 tablespoon white sugar

1 teaspoon salt

¼ teaspoon ground pepper

1 bay leaf

½ cup half-and-half cream

In a large saucepan, sauté the garlic in butter for 1 to 2 minutes. Stir in flour until blended, then slowly add chicken broth. Stir in tomato paste until well blended.

Stir in sugar and salt and pepper. Add the bay leaf.

Bring everything to a boil, cooking and stirring for 5 minutes, until thickened. Reduce heat and slowly stir in cream. Let simmer for 3 to 5 minutes. Remove bay leaf. Serve.

• OLD RELIABLE LENTIL SOUP •

TOTAL TIME: 60 MINUTES

SERVINGS: 8

300 CALORIES

1 ½ cups red lentils, rinsed
2 celery stalks, chopped
½ onion, chopped
1 medium carrot, peeled and chopped
1 teaspoon dried oregano
½ cup brown or white rice
½ cup fresh parsley leaves, chopped
1 cup chopped tomatoes
10 cups vegetable or chicken stock
Salt and pepper to taste

Combine all ingredients in a large soup pot. Bring to a boil, then reduce heat to low. Cover pot and cook for 45 minutes or until lentils are soft. Adjust salt and pepper to taste and serve.

• CHIPPER CHAPPER CHICKPEA SOUP •

TOTAL TIME: 40 MINUTES

SERVINGS: 4

UNDER 200 CALORIES

1 tablespoon olive oil	½ teaspoon dried basil
1 onion, chopped	One 15-ounce can tomato sauce
1 clove garlic, peeled and minced	One 15-ounce can chickpeas
2 celery stalks, chopped	½ teaspoon dried oregano
1 green bell pepper, chopped	½ teaspoon dried parsley
2 teaspoons rosemary leaves, finely chopped	4 cups water
	Salt and pepper to taste

Heat olive oil in a large saucepan over medium heat. Add onion, garlic, celery, green pepper, rosemary, and basil. Sauté for approximately 5 minutes or until onions are tender.

Add tomato sauce, chickpeas, oregano, parsley, and water. Reduce heat to low, cover, and let simmer for 30 minutes. Season with salt and pepper to taste. Serve.

Optional: Purée half of the soup in a blender until smooth, then return to the chunky soup.

• COURAGEOUS CARROT SOUP •

TOTAL TIME: 40 MINUTES

SERVINGS: 4

UNDER 200 CALORIES

2 tablespoons sweet cream
   butter
1 large onion, chopped
2½ cups diced carrots
½ teaspoon grated fresh
   gingerroot
2 cups vegetable or chicken
broth
1 cup water
2 tablespoons chopped
   fresh dill
½ cup heavy whipping cream
Salt and pepper to taste
¼ cup sour cream

Melt butter in a medium saucepan. Add onion and cook in covered saucepan on low heat for 20 minutes. Add carrots, ginger, broth, water, and dill, then bring to a boil. Reduce heat, and simmer until carrots are tender when pierced.

Remove the saucepan from heat and carefully transfer soup to a blender. Start by using the pulse mode on the blender, then increase speed and purée until smooth.

Return the soup to the saucepan and add cream, stirring over high heat until hot (do not bring to a boil).

Add salt and pepper to taste. Top with sour cream. Serve.

• BONE-HUGGIN' BEEF STEW •

TOTAL TIME: 1½ HOURS

SERVINGS: 6

300 CALORIES

2 pounds boneless beef
chuck roast, cut into
1-inch cubes

3 tablespoons flour

2 tablespoons vegetable oil

2 yellow onions, cut into
1-inch pieces

1 clove garlic, peeled and
minced

3 cups beef stock or broth

2 medium carrots, peeled

and chopped

2 stalks celery, cut into
1-inch pieces

1 bay leaf

¼ teaspoon dried rosemary

¼ teaspoon dried thyme

1 teaspoon salt

1 pound Yukon gold pota-
toes, peeled, cut into
large chunks

Pepper to taste

Coat beef with flour. Heat the oil in large heavy pot or Dutch
oven with tight-fitting lid on medium-high heat. Add the
beef, browning on all sides.

Once browned, remove the beef and place in bowl, leav-
ing excess oil and beef drippings in the pot. Lower heat to
medium. Add onions to the pot and sauté for approximately
5 minutes.

Add garlic and cook for 1 minute.

Add stock, carrots, celery, bay leaf, rosemary, thyme,
beef, and salt. Return the soup to a gentle simmer, cover, and
cook for approximately 40 minutes.

Add potatoes and simmer, covered, for 20 minutes.

Remove cover, raise heat to medium, and stir occasionally for 20 minutes or until meat and vegetables are tender. Remove bay leaf. Season to taste and serve.

If stew is too thick, adjust by adding more stock or water.

• SUCCULENT BUTTERNUT SQUASH SOUP •

TOTAL TIME: 60 MINUTES

SERVINGS: 6

UNDER 200 CALORIES

2 tablespoons unsalted
  butter

1 large onion, chopped

3 cups butternut squash,
  peeled, seeded, and
  cubed

1 Granny Smith apple,
  peeled, cored, and diced

1 cup carrots, peeled and
  diced

1 cup apple cider

3 cups low-sodium chicken
  broth

½ teaspoon chopped fresh
  thyme

½ cup light cream

¼ teaspoon ground nutmeg

1 teaspoon salt

¼ teaspoon freshly ground
  pepper

Melt the butter in a large pot over medium-high heat. Stir in onion and cook until soft, about 5 minutes. Add squash and apple and sauté for 5 minutes, or until beginning to soften.

Add carrots, cider, broth, thyme, and bring the mixture to a boil. Reduce heat to simmer, cover, and cook until squash and carrots are tender, approximately 15 to 20 minutes.

Carefully purée the soup in small batches in a blender. Once entire soup is puréed, return to the pot and stir in the cream. Season with nutmeg, salt, and pepper. Let simmer for approximately 5 minutes, then serve.

• GAZPACHO SOUP •

READY TIME: 30 MINUTES (NOT INCLUDING CHILLING)

SERVINGS: 4

UNDER 200 CALORIES

3 tomatoes, chopped

1 large cucumber, peeled and chopped

½ red onion, chopped

1 yellow pepper, chopped

1 clove garlic, peeled and minced

1 celery stalk, chopped

1 tablespoon extra-virgin olive oil

2 tablespoons wine vinegar

2 tablespoons lemon juice

3 cups vegetable cocktail juice

Combine all ingredients in large glass bowl and mix. Cover and refrigerate for at least 3 hours to allow the flavors to blend. Serve chilled.

Index